HOOKUP
WITHOUT
HEARTBREAK

HOOKUP WITHOUT HEARTBREAK

How to feel empowered
after casual sex

Lia Holmgren

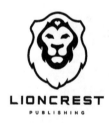

LIONCREST
PUBLISHING

HOOKUP WITHOUT HEARTBREAK
How to Feel Empowered after Casual Sex

ISBN 978-1-5445-0159-8 *Paperback*
        978-1-5445-0160-4 *Ebook*

HUMANS CAN

TURN SUFFERING

INTO ART.

CONTENTS

DISCLAIMER

. . . .

Before you start reading this book, I want you to understand my view of casual sex and hookups[1]: while I consider them fantastic entertainment and generally healthy outlets for our sexual desires, they also pose a risk of us getting hurt. At the end of the day, I'm not advocating for casual sex, nor am I against it. That said, it's part of our culture. So, **I created this guide for women who enjoy casual sex and want to learn how to best navigate the days after without feeling hurt.** Here, I share my hard-learned lessons to give my fellow females tips on how to overcome any soul pain they might experience after participating in a casual hookup.

---

[1] The American Psychological Association defines hookups as brief, uncommitted sexual encounters between individuals who are not romantic partners or dating each other. Garcia et al. define hookup as "a single act involving sexual intimacy such as kissing, touching, petting, or intercourse between two people who are friends or strangers, that lasts one night without the expectation of developing a relationship."

Justin R. Garcia, Chris Reiber, Sean G. Massey, and Ann M. Merriwether, "Sexual Hookup Culture: A Review," 16, no. 2 (June 2012): 161–76, https://doi.org/10.1037/a0027911.

This book sheds a light on the different sexual behaviors between men and women. Here's what you can expect:

FOR WOMEN

"I'm a slut and no man will want to marry me."

"I'm going to stay alone because men are scared of me."

"I'm too independent and powerful, and men like subordinate girls."

"All men cheat."

Have you ever told yourself any of these things?

I have. For years, I was figuring out the formula for enjoying sex for what it is, without the noise of shame, judgment, and slut-shaming that is so prevalent in our society. When I was younger and got hurt, going out, partying, and drinking was the ultimate "letting go" recipe for my broken heart. Now I know this behavior leads nowhere, and I advocate for conscious self-care and self-love instead. I want you to read this book to save yourself from unnecessary trauma. Even a small negative incident can traumatize your brain and create limiting beliefs about yourself and men in general—like the ones listed above.

None of these limiting beliefs is true, but whatever you believe can create your reality, which can further negatively affect your love and dating life. This book will help you to un-fuck yourself.

The new me knows that there are grown and self-confident men who don't cheat, who like independent and powerful women, and who aren't scared of "sluts"—quite the opposite, they praise them.

Lastly, please remember that women are not the only ones who get hurt. Men also have a fair share of disappointments with their casual sex partners. The difference is that most men can deal with this situation more easily and move on much faster.

In this book, I will tell you a few stories I heard from my work as a relationship and intimacy coach and help you overcome the double standard around sexuality in our culture. Why? So you can decide what approach to sex works best for you and prepare for the next hookup.

Content created for women resides in Chapters 1–3, but I'm sure you'll be curious about the last "For Men" part as well.

FOR MEN

I want you to know that I'm not a man-hater and this book isn't full of blame and men-shaming. Quite the opposite; I love men, and I couldn't imagine my life without them. I never was a girly girl, and in most of my personal and professional settings, guys surround me. I used to think I knew how they think, what tricks to use to make them do what I want, and what turns them on or off. I believed I had it all figured out and that I couldn't get hurt ever again.

But I was wrong.

No matter how much I thought I knew men, life is full of surprises and sometimes brings you a particular kind of man who can quickly rock your world up and, much quicker, down.

If you are a man, keep reading so you can learn more about what's happening in a woman's mind after a hookup. Or skip ahead to the section, which covers useful steps for how you can help her feel better, even if you have no interest in seeing her again. A text message doesn't cost much, and it can make a world of difference. Unless you are an egotist who thrives on female suffering, I think you should pay attention to those few pages. Thank you—the Queendom will appreciate you.

For real enjoyment, I suggest you read Chapter 3, which will provide information on the history of human sexual behaviors and why women act differently than men around sex, and Chapter 4, which is created to help you get out of a messy situation. If you're very curious, feel free to read all the chapters, as I believe that many of the twenty-four tips are useful not only for women.

NOTE ON CONFIDENTIALITY

The names of the interviewees and participants in the stories have been changed to ensure discretion.

INTRODUCTION

· ·

"*I can't believe I did it again*. I feel like a complete fool!" Amber said through tears in our coaching session. "This wasn't my first rodeo, and I really thought I was already immune and knew how to compartmentalize casual sex from love. I knew he was just a fling, yet here I am, longing for more! He totally possessed my mind," she sobbed.

As I compassionately listened to her share her story, I nodded softly. I'd been there too, and not only once.

After they met at a corporate dinner, Mr. Charmer reached out to Amber multiple times suggesting a friendly drink or coffee. "I was super attracted to him from day one, but I wasn't sure I wanted to go there. We were tight in a professional relationship, and my workload and personal engagements didn't allow me to take him up on his offer for months. But then when we finally met, after hours of talking and flirting, I knew I wanted him. I was ready to initiate a

1

sexual encounter. I made it clear that I was interested, and our texting that night quickly shifted to sexting. He sent me sexy texts about me being in an Italian villa, walking barefoot on the cold floor, making my way to the bedroom. I sent him my own erotic imagination in another message."

After weeks of planning, they met for the third time. It was a proper rendezvous, starting with an elegant dinner and drinks that led to a passionate night full of sex.

"I really enjoyed his company and the conversation, and then the sex was incredible. I haven't felt connected like that with someone in a long time. Although we barely knew each other, he was making love to me. He even said that he felt close to me and comfortable around me, like he had known me for a long time. The feeling was mutual. To my surprise, he spent the night too! Most first-timers would leave right after they cum. I really hoped to see him again."

Amber kept describing the story, and I could see tears in her eyes as she stared at the wall of my office. "I'm honestly surprised that he never asked to meet up again."

"So, he never reached out at all?" I asked, feeling for this woman and knowing what she was going through all too well.

"Besides a 'Thank you for a wonderful time' and 'How are you feeling?' messages the day after, I haven't heard anything else. Not a peep."

I tried to soothe her. "I know how you feel, Amber, but there is no point in blaming him or yourself."

"I know, Lia. I'm not making myself a victim. I'm an adult woman, and we both wanted to play. I have been thinking it through for weeks. But still, this shit hurts!"

"What makes you the most upset?" I asked, wondering what she would like to hear so she could let go sooner. "How could he make you feel better?"

"He just disappeared from the world—hasn't even reached out to meet for tea or given me a phone call for closure. I don't expect men to marry me right after," she said, and smiled for the first time, "but not knowing what happened, especially when there were months of texts prior to this experience, drives me nuts."

Amber believed that closure would give her peace of mind—something she desperately desired—freedom from the feeling of maniacally checking her phone every thirty minutes. "I just want to move on with my life!" she said, a flash of anger in her eyes.

Amber's story illustrates a common problem in the Queendom: no matter how many sexual partners we've had, how experienced we are, or how sure we are that it will just be a casual encounter, we often get attached. The reasons originate in nature and nurture, as I will get into in the later chapters of this book, but the point is clear: women struggle more than men to process casual hookup experiences. After having sex with , everything changes. You become infatuated and are flooded with feelings and emotions for days and sometimes weeks after. You think about . You wonder if he liked it and if you're going to see him again. You're checking your phone, hoping for at least a little beep or a social media like from. He's everywhere—in your mind and your conversations. You crave and want more. It's like a drug that has been taken away from an addict!

Wouldn't it be perfect to enjoy sex for what it is and move on without any of the above thoughts? The worst part is that post-sex energy is often the opposite on his end: while your interest in him skyrockets, his interest in you wanes right after you sleep with him! The curves on the graph suddenly go in opposite directions, which leaves you uncomfortable and confused.

After talking to hundreds of women of all ages, in all positions, from all walks of life, I have rarely met a woman who is able to simply move on with her day after a one-night stand like nothing ever happened—a woman who can compartmentalize and focus on work and friends. Most of them shared the same anxiety about the unknown. I can sympathize with them because I'm one of them. Trust me, I love hookups, but I too often got hurt and needed to practice different mindfulness techniques and visit my favorite psychotherapist to get over !

After many years of hookup experiences, I found techniques that work magic and could make my hookup experiences beautiful and manageable. Today, I feel a strong responsibility to guide other women, to show them how to feel empowered after casual sex!

Are you one of the few ladies who already have this all figured out and enjoy men for the sake of pleasure and their cocks? Lucky you! I envy you and really want to know some of your tricks! Please share them with me at my email, liaholmgren@protonmail.com, so I can anonymously post them on my blog for other ladies to learn from.

WHY SHOULD YOU TRUST ME?

My story began in communist Czechoslovakia, a rigid, cookie-cutter environment where sex was never openly discussed. When I was eleven years old, the avalanche of puberty ushered in a new awakening, one that nobody had prepared me for, and I became an exceptionally horny teenager. I kissed and licked the metal doorframe next to my bed every single night before I went to sleep, imagining it was a boyfriend. I masturbated with books, bed frames, and my hand. At some point, I tried to handcuff myself to the bed and managed to drop the key from the bed to the floor. My grandma came in and found me crying, then promptly broke the key in the lock. We would have had to call the fire department if my granddad hadn't been handy and able to get me out of them. The experience left me with red marks on my wrists—and as you can surely imagine, a massive sense of embarrassment.

I spent my teenage years fantasizing about sex and learning what makes my body feel good. Soon after, I began to explore with both men and women. I created my own hookup culture in the strict and reserved post-communistic country where "sluts" were shamed and excluded from society. I was proud to be sexually adventurous—a so-called slut—and couldn't understand why, as a woman, I was not allowed to get pleasure—and when I did, I was shamed by others. But no matter how many "defeats" I suffered, they never shook my confidence. Although it was difficult, this attitude allowed me to keep gathering many interesting sexual experiences. In between my longer-term relationships, I always gladly returned to the hobby of hooking up, where I had a lot of fun accompanied by a lot of psychological pain. I cried for men more than I probably should have, and I often wished that someone would give me a recipe for how to manage my feelings after casual encounters.

From the time I was a teenager, my life has been very interesting. I have lived and loved in eight countries and traveled to over fifty. I have collected my fair share of experiences when it comes to men and dating—all of which have helped me become the strong, confident woman I am today.

In addition to my wide range of sexual experiences, I spent over seven years studying psychology, biology, nutrition, hypnosis, life coaching, meditation, negotiation strategies, and conflict resolution. While I was studying, I spent ten years working as a professional dominatrix and later on, as an intimacy and relationship coach helping individuals and couples navigate topics around sex, communication, and love.

Throughout my studies and research, I read tons of papers in sociology and neuroscience, from which I will provide you with the most interesting findings. The goal of my studies was to understand every aspect of the human body and mind when it comes to sex, and the interaction between the two.

While writing this book, my curiosity took over and I had to interview men about casual sex and why they act the way they do after a hookup. Fifty kind men, between the ages of twenty-five and fifty-five, shared their dirty little secrets and truths about how they think, feel, and act around hookups. I wanted to know how they get out of an awkward situation, what they say when they do want to see her again, and if they have any aftercare or post-hookup rules. I will include those details throughout the book.

Let's begin!

Part 1

· ·

HOW TO PROTECT YOUR HEART

Today, the media talks about the clitoris as if it were the biggest discovery of the last century and mentions hookups with the same frequency as tips on where to get new shoes. Well-known cosmetic companies market and sell beauty products to women through slogans that state, "hookup perfect." The movement of modern-day women's sexual liberation is real—and, clearly, highly marketable.

It's so real, in fact, that often, millennials and younger generations are so busy hustling from partner to partner that traditional techniques —one in which the man approaches the woman in a lengthy courtship

—seem antiquated. Maybe even boring. Why do all that work when, through dating apps, the perfect lover might be just one click away? Due to career growth and busy social lives, the old "play hard to get" technique isn't feasible—or fun—for many women anymore. Men know this, and many expect hookups to be the only thing they are ready for "at the beginning." The truth is that we live in a fast world and want instant gratification.

So where is the problem? Mutually agreed upon casual sex seems to be freeing, empowering, and so much fun! And it is! Sex is wonderful when done right, and connecting with another human being on an intimate level is crucial for our well-being.

Yet, we know the pleasure of a one-night stand can quickly turn into torture when we become attached against our will. And although sometimes pleasure and pain go hand in hand, this is the kind of psychological pain that shouldn't be part of our experience.

In the times of my misery and mental discomfort caused by being ignored and disregarded after hookups, I decided to observe my mind and emotions to see what was actually going on. I paid close attention to my thoughts and saw that my mood shifted depending on the stories I told myself. My feelings after a hookup went awry, ranging from awkwardness, confusion, humiliation, regret, anger, sadness, anxiety, and self-pity to emptiness, shame, and guilt.

I realized that I must shift them toward positive ones. Easier said than done, right? Don't worry. Here, I've broken my insights down into the twenty-four tips you need to survive in the modern hookup culture.

Tip #1:
EVALUATE BEFORE YOU HOOK UP

You meet him and like him, you exchange numbers and share some messages. He is reaching out to you, and you can read between the lines: he's interested... in fucking you. While having drinks, you gaze deep into each other's eyes, and you feel a familiar, sexy warmth all over your body. You agree to see him again very soon. You get so turned on by the fantasy of having sex with him that, back home, you take your favorite toy and masturbate while thinking of him.

Or, perhaps you are horny, lonely, and decide to join one of the quick and easy "dating" apps. As you swipe right and left, you're not looking for a boyfriend—you're looking for who might be around to "cuddle."

The scenarios for how to meet someone for sex vary, but the ultimate goal is to have fun and bond with another human being that you're attracted to. The main purpose of sex nowadays is pleasure and connection, and seldom procreation. This makes the decision about with whom to have sex or not much easier—but even then, it's important to consider all aspects of the hookup up front.

Why? Because by making informed decisions, you can protect yourself from being hurt and feeling like crap afterward. The most important questions to ask yourself before your encounter are: "What is my intention with this person? What am I fantasizing about, and what do I crave?" Are you looking for sexual pleasure? Do you want a friend with benefits? Are you looking for dating or a casual lover? Are you looking for a long-term partner, as your heart craves romance? Or is your head not there yet, and all you want is to get laid?

It is really important to know and be honest with yourself. Once you know the answers, you can pick the right approach and feel good about it later. If you want sexual pleasure only, don't wait—go for it. If you're looking for more commitment, I recommend you take a slower approach to sex. Even if he seems impatient, let him wait. If he's like most men, he likes the challenge.

Sadly, even in times of female sexual liberation, many men disrespect women who like casual sex and have sex with a stranger too quickly. It's an ugly double standard, and I will talk more about it in the later chapters of this book. So, if you have a fantasy of marriage or a prince on a white horse, quickly hooking up is a bad idea. (Already slept with him? Don't worry! There are always exceptions to the rule, and some hookups will turn into relationships. According to one survey,[2] 11 percent of the participants ended up in a casual romantic

---

[2] Eliza M. Weitbrecht and Sarah W. Whitton, "Expected, Ideal, and Actual Relational Outcomes of Emerging Adults' 'Hook Ups,'" *Personal Relationships* 24, no. 4 (November 21, 2017): 902–16, https://doi.org/10.1111/pere.12220.

relationship and another 12 percent in committed monogamous relationships.)

Personally, all my relationships stemmed from casual hookups. I had no patience to wait because I've always been a particularly horny person, so sex on the first or second date was a norm. Another reason for this was that I don't like bad surprises. Can you imagine waiting in anticipation for two months, falling in love with his looks and personality, only to discover that you don't fit with the size and shape of his cock, or that he is a clumsy lover? Ouch—what a waste of time that would be.

The last and most important question to ask yourself before you hook up is: are you ready to take the risk that he will have sex with you and never talk to you again? If you don't care about that, then have fun!

But if you thought you wouldn't give a fuck, and then did, read further—I have more tips to help you get over it.

Tip #2:
CONDOMS AND BOUNDARIES

You decided to hook up, and you're positive that you won't get attached. Great, I'm with you! In this section, I want to make sure you're taking some basic precautions and establishing your boundaries.

First, for your first date, make sure you're safe. I don't want this book to be a manual on how to get laid safely, and I'm sure you know many of these things, but I really have to mention it here. I care about you and repetition ensures you won't forget about it, in spite of oxytocin tra-la-la-land.

First, find out as much as you can about him, including where he works. Check his social media to see if you have mutual friends. If you trust some of them, don't worry about asking for references. Preferably, let some of your friends know where you'll be and with whom. If it's his place or your place, make sure you're safe. I wouldn't travel to a mountain cabin on a first date.

And **bring condoms!** Don't let this task be his responsibility, because you don't know him. Choose the ones you like to use and have them ready. STIs will be one less thing to worry about afterward.

Next, it's time to think about your boundaries for the encounter. How do you set them? Try this: think about the act in detail. Imagine how it will make you feel to lie naked and spread your legs for him. Does it feel sexy and comfortable? What about it feels sexy? Him holding you? Him kissing you? Or him fucking you hard? Perhaps you really want to relax and let him please you orally. Think about this soberly and figure out what kind of physical connection you are comfortable with.

Before you meet him for drinks, make sure you give yourself a clear YES and write down your personal disclaimer. Something along these lines: "I know that this might be just a one-time thing, and there is a chance that he is only being charming and sweet so he can get laid. I have no expectations of him texting me, calling me, or wanting to see me again. I'm accepting this as an experience that I chose to have in my life, and I'm OK with whatever comes after. My intention is to get properly laid, fulfill my fantasy of being a [insert whatever pleases you], and let him give me at least one orgasm so I can feel rejuvenated and fulfilled afterward." Repeat this loudly so it stays engraved in your mind. And write it down on a sticky note.

Once you establish your boundaries, communicate them at the right time. Of course, you don't want to call him before your rendezvous and shout at him, "I'm definitely not going to fuck you tomorrow night," or "You can only taste my pussy and suck on my nipples, honey." That would definitely ruin the mystery and take the fun away from your first play date.

A bad idea is to wait to tell him about your boundaries until after three glasses of wine at dinner, because by then, you might be tipsy and uncontrollably horny. You might be thinking: "Boundaries? What boundaries?" or "I'll see how the night goes…" No, you won't see, you already know that you will end up in bed with him, and you might be upset about your drunk decision the next day. "Here we go! I acted like a slut again!" I can hear you calling.

But you also don't want to wait until the point of no return—you, lying naked on his sofa, trying to turn back time and say you only wanted a kiss. That's a perfect recipe for a frustrating night. But even then, remember this: **there is always a way back, and nobody can pressure you to do things you aren't comfortable with. Just because you're naked doesn't mean you have to fuck him!**

If you need a tip to get out of it elegantly, pull the goddess move: tell him that first you'd like to cum with his tongue. It's a rather difficult task to accomplish on the first date. If he can't make you cum, tell him that it means you need more time to get comfortable and closer with him to be able to reach orgasm, so you'd like to postpone the penetrative sex.

Say you've communicated your boundaries properly, and the night has been a success for both of you, on your own terms. Do you remember that disclaimer you wrote down? Look at it first thing when you wake up, satisfied, with your sexy JBF (just been fucked) hair.

Tip #3:
ONLY FANTASIZE ABOUT THE SEX

You're about to see him in a couple of days. It's been a while since you met and started flirting. The idea of having sex with him was born some weeks ago, and you agreed to meet for a date night. Sake and sushi at a sexy restaurant? Hell yes! Perhaps one more cocktail in a jazz bar afterward? It will be a great night.

You arrange for a manicure, pedicure, and blowout in preparation …not to mention spending hours planning your outfit. You might even buy some new lingerie for the occasion. You feel giddy. Excited.

Until the emotions shift.

Suddenly, you start to fantasize about him taking you on a vacation this summer. You could practice tennis with him every Sunday, right? He said he's a good player. Maybe he can show you his weekend cabin in the mountains, which he mentioned. *When was his birthday again? you think, your brain having gone off the rails. I need to ask! What could I get him?*

OK, stop right there.

Your fantasies with this man should center on the sexual experience you're about to have with him. This is healthy because the anticipation will make you more turned on—which leads to a more satisfying sexual experience. How will his cock look? How is his touch as a lover? How might his kiss feel on your skin?

The future, though? No fantasies about that. Your thoughts about vacations, an ongoing texting romance, elegant dinners, and how you will introduce him to your friends and family are out of place.

I'm being real with you for a reason: to protect you from major disappointment. You really have no idea what will follow your rendezvous.

Trust me. As Dr. Dispenza,[3] my favorite neuroscientist, says, when we are focused on visualizing—which I also call fantasizing—and paying attention to all the details of the scenario, our brains can't distinguish between real experiences and imagined experiences. That means your brain can believe your visualization and store the experience of it as a memory. If things turn out otherwise, the disappointment will be much greater.

Let me explain in detail. The fact is that you don't know this man. You shared some texts, he invited you for a drink or dinner, and it's obvious that he wants to have sex with you. And you want to have sex with him. That's where it ends. Nothing less, nothing more. Thinking about him in a capacity outside the bedroom creates a feeling of a serious relationship that only exists in your head. Once he is gone from your life, you will feel sad for this stranger as if he had been your boyfriend. I know it sounds crazy, but that's how our brains work. How could you be sad if someone loses interest in you after a one-night stand if you barely know him all along?

---

[3] Joe Dispenza, *Becoming Supernatural: How Common People are Doing the Uncommon* (Carlsbad, CA: Hay House, 2017).

Tip #4:
TWO DRINKS MAXIMUM

To play with someone you just met can understandably be scary. You may feel self-conscious, especially at the prospect of getting naked and intimate with someone new if this is outside of your comfort zone.

To "loosen up," it's common for women (and men) to turn to alcohol to rid themselves of inhibitions and performance anxiety.

I do not advocate for the route of intoxication with drugs or alcohol. As women, we can become sloppy sooner than we realize. Not only is that unsexy, but it plays against our orgasms.

It's true! Orgasms become more difficult to reach when we are under the influence of alcohol. One glass or two is fine, but we all have limits. Know yours. If you don't, you might agree to do things you normally wouldn't do, such as having unprotected or anal sex. You don't want to wake up with a pain in your butt, literally, or with two guys instead of one. You might also agree to take drugs that could negatively interact with alcohol, such as ketamine or GHB. Then, not only are you not going to enjoy the sex, but also, you're putting your life at risk.

And what if he wants to play the Houdini[4] game with you? What the hell is Houdini, you might ask? Well, here is an Urban Dictionary definition for you: "You are doing a girl doggy style whilst she is facing a window to the outdoors...halfway thru your thrusting, you do a pullout move (to say finger her a little) but then your friend who is strategically hidden in the room sneaks in and inserts himself as if it were you. This is when you quietly exit the room, reappearing outside the window when you—now smiling ear to ear—wave at your girl, who comes to the realization that, 'if he is out there, who is fucking me?'"

I'm telling you, weird shit can happen. Keep your mind sober, have fun, and you will be just fine.

But wait—what if *he's* drinking like a fish? It could be an honest mistake. Or it could be that he is (a) super insecure and needs to drink a lot in order to fuck, or (b) an alcoholic. You don't want that either, especially because he might become more aggressive and less attentive to your needs when he is drunk. And you came into this with the desire to cum, right? That's not going to happen if either of you is three sheets to the wind.

If you see him drinking too much, excuse yourself by telling him you have a headache and need to go home. Notice his reaction when you

---

[4] "the houdini," Urban Dictionary, accessed May 12, 2021, https://www.urbandictionary.com/define.php?term=the%20houdini.

announce that you're going to leave. Is he understanding, or does he act angry and needy? It's an overall good test!

Tip #5:
BE THE GODDESS. LET HIM PLEASE YOU.

What should you wear on your first date? What should you cook for him? What lingerie should you wear to look hot? How could you give a better blowjob?

I remember growing up reading teenage girls' magazines such as *Cosmo Girl, Seventeen*, etc. Most of the advice was based on one thing: how to please men. Sadly, without knowing better, I followed these idiotic ideas and became a puppet for men. All I wanted to achieve was to give my lovers a great time and for them to like me. When they never called me again, I was devastated, wondering what I could have done better and what I had done wrong. My self-esteem often suffered, but I was too young to understand the harmful effect of this "pleasing" trend. After many sexual partners, I was still wondering when I would experience the great pleasure they were talking about in the magazine. I liked exploring, but the only orgasm I could reach was with masturbation. Thankfully, at least that reassured me that there was nothing wrong with my body!

I've spent years exploring the opposite of those bullshit headlines and asking a key question: what about female pleasure? Unfortunately, even today, I don't know of many quality articles teaching men how to please women the right way. When I find some tips, they are lousy and more entertaining than useful, like... "Make a move in the shape of a figure eight around her clit!" Really? I first came from a clitoral orgasm with a man when I was nineteen, after being sexually active for over four years. I had to rub myself on his pubic bone in the un-sexiest position. I will never forget how weirdly he stared at me, probably wondering what the hell I was doing.

All the acrobatic stuff that guys wanted to do with me was more painful than fun, but I thought it was supposed to be that way. The worst part was that all the lame advice made me feel ashamed to ask men to please me. I didn't want to "bother" them with my requests.

Thankfully, that has changed, mainly through my work as a dominatrix. After meeting many men from all walks of life, I realized that their biggest desire is female pleasure. Most men want to see the woman happy and satisfied. They're struggling to find the right pleasure buttons without proper guidance. They're shy to ask because they don't want to come across as creepy or inexperienced. They want to be good lovers, but many don't know how. Women, by default, do not ask for pleasure or give directions. The worst is when they even fake orgasms, leaving the man with the impression that he's done well...just to get more of what didn't work.

I was shocked to hear many married and divorced men telling me that they never had sexual conversations with their partners and—

sometimes even after decades of marriage—didn't know what their partners liked. That's why they came to me. What they expected from a dominatrix was to lead. To tell them what I liked and wanted. To command them.

Although there was a certain amount of sexual fantasy and dirty talk, as a dominatrix, I didn't have direct sexual contact with clients. Usually, I did command my submissive clients to massage my feet, kiss my boots, and massage my shoulders, and I spanked them in return. They loved to see me taking the initiative. Domination allowed me to reclaim my power and self-esteem.

Dear ladies, communicate and navigate. The man you are about to play with is super horny, like every other dude. He wants to get laid and will be "into" you no matter what. There is no rocket science to male orgasm, and men cum more easily than women. A study[5] in which researchers surveyed 12,295 participants, showed that only 10 percent of women reach orgasm in a casual hookup encounter, and only 19 percent of women, as opposed to 55 percent of men, receive oral sex during a first-time hookup.

Raise this number and put your pleasure ahead of his. You don't need to work too hard to impress him with your porn-star performance. (Sure, if you'd *like* to deep-throat him, go for it, but only if you're really

---

[5] Elizabeth A. Armstrong, Paula England, and Alison C. K. Fogarty, "Accounting for Women's Orgasm and Sexual Enjoyment in College Hookups and Relationships," *American Sociological Review* 77, no. 3 (May 7, 2012): 435–62, https://doi.org/10.1177/0003122412445802.

into it!) The key is to be yourself—show him the things you enjoy and how you enjoy them. Let him worship your body. If you enjoy getting oral sex, ask him to please you that way. There's no shame in receiving pleasure, and my favorite rule that I heard from a close friend years ago is, "Before a man enters your temple, tell him it must be well eaten!"

Trust me, men love to be led and shown what women like in bed, and the true gentleman appreciates the woman's orgasm more than his own anyway. It's almost like getting a massage. You most likely won't find it difficult to tell the masseur where s/he should press harder and where it feels good, so this is the same principle. Enjoy, goddess!

Tip #6:
SEX SHOULD BE AN ACT OF LOVE, EVEN IF IT'S CASUAL!

You may be thinking, *Wait, Lia. I thought we were talking about protecting my heart in a hookup. Why are you mentioning love?*

Here's why: if we are making love to someone and creating a deeply connected experience, it will allow us to cope with the aftermath of this hookup better. To be fucked like a whore and never texted again feels terrible. To have a great and loving experience with someone might make us miss that person more, but we will feel better about ourselves. If he never texts or calls, you won't feel like he took advantage of you and disappeared.

But how can you make love to someone you barely know? You don't want to sound needy. One of the hardest things for us humans is to show vulnerability of any kind. That's why men often stay away from soft and gentle sex. They want to fuck hard, so they don't look like less of a man. Many men feel ashamed to need intimacy and connection. Women are also scared to ask for more tenderness and more intimate sex for the same reasons, so they tolerate unenjoyable sex. It's a sad dynamic because we all crave intimacy, love, and connection.

It's fine to be romantic, gentle, and express compliments to a casual lover. There are no rules on how hard or soft sex can be. Do whatever suits you. It's fine to make love to each other like you've known each other for a long time. Passion and connection make sex better. Even if you have many lovers on rotation, every one of them should be treated with respect and appreciation, and the same treatment is important for you. Give and receive. Our hearts are big enough, and we can share love with other human beings even without being in committed, long-term relationships. It's about the love that you have for someone *in the moment*; what was before or what will be after is unimportant.

I'm a big believer in having the best sex possible, an act that will blow your mind and that you will remember forever. Life is too short to have lousy sex, and after many years of experimenting, I can surely state that nothing is better than lovemaking! It feels like dropping an incredible ecstasy pill.

So how to make love with a stranger, you might ask?

Communicate your needs as you play. If you feel like he is trying to impress you or treat you more as a whore than a lover, stop him. Say, "Did I do something bad to you to make you fuck me like this?" and giggle. I have used that sentence many times before, and it worked. In their desire to "perform," men often forget to be loving and they only focus on (their) climax. Isn't it annoying when a man says while he's fucking you, "Are you close?" or "I want you to come, baby!" Gosh, for me it's a real buzz kill. I feel so pressured that I won't come at all. On the flip side, I know this works for men! Telling him, "Cum for me, baby! Give me a big load on my tits!" will definitely do the trick when you have had enough and want him to finish. But it's not the same for us women.

Instead, tell him to look into your eyes. Tell him to breathe deeply with you. Good breath technique while having sex makes the whole act more intense, and you will have a stellar orgasm. And the bonus is that it will make him last longer. Exchange dirty talk for some soft and sexy sentences. Dirty talk can be fun for a bit, but not over the entire sexual experience. You don't want to tell him you love him —that would be really awkward—but "I love the way you hold my hips!" sounds sexy.

Be fully present. The experience is so much better than thinking of other people or having your mind wander. You can think of others when you're masturbating or when you're in a long-term relationship and need a bit of refreshment. A hookup, though, is not the time.

A warning that's important here: do not confuse passion with love. This can happen due to oxytocin, a hormone and neurotransmitter that is released when, for example, we're hugging, kissing, and having sex. It makes us feel like we're in love. Women have much higher levels of oxytocin than men, and its effect is much stronger. This can come in handy when giving birth and bonding with a child. It also has other health benefits, but the downside is that it might make you feel in love with the man you just had sex with (whom you barely know). Next time, when you feel out of control and want to marry and have babies with your one-night stand, remember: it's all oxytocin's fault.

Tip #7:
TEST THE WATERS

Picture this: a woman wakes up groggily, the sun shining on her face through poorly closed curtains. "Ouch, my head hurts! Why is there so much light? What's the time?" she thinks, trying to find her cell phone on the nightstand. Moving her hand around the bed, grabbing all sorts of things, it hits her: this isn't her home.

It starts coming back now. She realizes that she is naked, hungover, and there is a cute man lying next to her. She can only see his back, but she remembers the hot night they had. *Shit—I wanted to go home, and I must have fallen asleep*, she thinks.

She walks out of the bedroom and tries to find her belongings in the bundle of shoes and clothing lying in a line leading from the bedroom to the living room. The beginning of the line consists of her panties and stockings mixed with his jeans and a couple of used condoms. *Ugh.* She walks farther and finds her skirt and her heels. Her bra and blouse are the last items to be found on the sofa. Once she is dressed, she wants to leave without having to say goodbye. Her lover is already up, just stretching his arms and yawning. "Hi Sexy, did you find everything?"

"Yes, thank you! I'll go now. Have to get to work at some point," she says, kissing him quickly on his cheeks.

"Have a good day! That was fun!" he says with a mischievous smile as he turns to walk back to the bedroom.

After the woman leaves the man's house, days pass. She doesn't hear from him at all. No *Hello, how are you*? No *Thank you for the fun. You were really good the other night.* Not even a *Did you get home safe?*

All that... after giving him her vagina! What should she do now, she wonders?

This scenario is all too common. When it comes to follow-up policies, though, there isn't really a common answer on etiquette. So, I asked men about their follow-up policies. Seventy percent said they would definitely reach out if they wanted to see the woman again. The ones who wouldn't said that sometimes they get carried away with work and forget to reach out. You might think they lack proper etiquette, but in truth, some men disclosed that they don't reach out because they want the woman to be the first one to do so. That way, they can be sure the woman liked them. Some men are scared of rejection.

There are those men who like to play games. They want to keep a little bit of mystery around themselves and let the woman feel insecure about whether they liked her. They're playing something similar to the hot and cold game in seduction, which was well described by Robert Greene in the book Art of Seduction.[6] Perhaps you fucked his brains out, so he still needs to collect them in order to write.

We can think of many reasons, to the point that we waste time overthinking. So, let's get to the real question: what can you do if you can't get him out of your head?

Take action before you drive yourself completely crazy waiting for his message another week. Text him. We have freedom of expression, and the idea of being a good girl and having him reach out first is outdated. Remember, the goal of this guide is to help you calm your mind and protect your heart, not follow ridiculous societal rules.

For most romantics, including me, it would be nice to hear from him first, but if you are curious and want to test the waters, here is the

---

[6] Robert Greene, *The Art of Seduction* (London: Penguin Books, 2003),

plan: you can tell him how he made you feel in the twenty-four to forty-eight hours following the hookup. Keep the text simple. Let him know how much you liked the time that you spent together, that the sex was fun (for your sake, I hope it was) and wish him a great day or weekend. Wait for a reply before you suggest another meeting. He might do it before you. An easy message with a compliment will keep it light. You will see his reaction, and it will leave him space for hunting and asking you out. If you make it too easy for him, there is a chance he will lose interest.

Of course, I have met plenty of men who found it sexy that I took charge and initiated, but not everyone is like that. Give space to start because you will have plenty of opportunities to initiate later if the two of you become regular hookup buddies or partners.

Tip #8:
COMMUNICATION IS THE KEY

This will be a longer section, but I believe in the magic of effective communication to avoid misunderstandings and conflicts. To help illustrate my point, I'll share a little story: My friend Ella was completely smitten by Mark. She had been with him for a couple of months before they finally met. "It was one of the best sexual experiences in my life," she said to me the day after the hookup, excited and giddy. "We had an insane connection! It's totally casual, but I think I rocked his world. I'm giving him about two or three days, and he will want to see me again," she added with a smile on her face.

A week later, I got a message from Ella: "Can you believe it? Still nothing! What should I do?"

"Just text him and tell him you want to see him again. Not a big deal," was my simple advice.

Ella sent him a picture of herself in a sexy outfit, drinking a glass of champagne. "I'm thinking of you. How is work treating you?" she wrote. His reply came at 9:30 p.m.: "Busy and tired." That was it. Nothing more, leaving Ella angry and frustrated, almost ashamed, all evening.

The next morning, he thanked her for thinking of him and asked her what her plans were for the weekend. Instead of bringing some clarity to this conversation, she became even more annoyed and answered, "Not sure, might go to a friend's birthday party!" A great small-talk conversation example that led absolutely nowhere.

There are many communication issues to address here. First of all, why text so late and ask about work if you want to be clear about missing him? His "Any plans for the weekend?" made things even more convoluted. Ella *should* have responded: "No plans yet, let's hang out and [get naughty, cozy, kinky, or whatever you liked last time]." Instead, she didn't want to make the first move, and apparently neither did he. They were dancing around each other without anyone suggesting a rendezvous.

But Ella didn't see it that way. "Why the hell is he interested in my weekend plans? He can ask me out instead!" she said to me, upset and confused.

Do you ever catch yourself reading his messages and saying, "WTF does he mean?" Or do you draw a quick conclusion that he is not interested or doesn't want to see you again?

Stop.

It's time for clarification. It's understandable that at the beginning, when you two just met, there was a lot of mystery about who you were and what your intentions were. Being too direct could have come across as unsexy, sure. But remember that your happiness is of utmost importance, and you must determine how much ambiguity is comfortable to you. If he's Mr. Mysterious and you're not sure what he means, ask him. Don't assume. If he's about to become your friend or a fuck buddy, you must train him to communicate the way you like.

Quality communication is important for long-term satisfaction. Misunderstandings and assumptions made between the lines can hurt those relationships. Especially nowadays, when the most common form of communication is online messaging, not being clear can create a perfect storm of confusion to the point that the parties stop talking to each other for good. Before you assume, clarify. Ask him what he meant, and also be clear about what you want. Use sentences such as "Yes, let's do it!" or "No, I prefer we go elsewhere" or "I want to see you next week; does that work for you?" Mumbling and sending unclear messages, hoping the other party will decode them, is ineffective.

If he still doesn't reach out after you've been patient for a while, remind yourself that he might be on the shier side. Not only that, but you can give it one more shot. Call him or text him and tell him you are thinking of him and want to see him again. Put the fear aside and be direct. In the end, what's the worst thing that can happen to you? He says "no." So what? You'll survive, and there are another approximately 3.9 billion men out there!

To me, the best-case scenario is that you know you'll want to see him again the night of. What to do then? Tell him before you go your separate ways. Hug him, look into his eyes, and compliment him for his performance and other things you want him to know that you like about him. Say, "You are smart, funny, and I like the way you made love to me! You would make a perfect hookup buddy!" Add a little giggle and flattery. Too much can come across as fake, but a little bit doesn't hurt. People love to feel good about themselves, and compliments will stroke his ego and make him feel like a superhero. The hookup will stimulate him physically and psychologically, and there's a stronger chance that he will see you again soon.

In person, you can also observe his body language and facial expressions, which are missing in online communication. Is he enthusiastic about a potential new date? Is his tone of voice pleasant or rather hesitant? Is he giving you compliments in return? Maybe invite him to reach out to you with a simple phrase like, "Don't be a stranger—reach out. It turns me on to hear from you." This way he gets a green light to text you in case he wouldn't feel confident enough to do it.

With this tactic, you have brought as much clarity around your situation as possible. Now you can let him reach out. Be patient, please. Everyone has their own texting style, seduction technique, and things to do in their daily lives, which might not necessarily synchronize with yours. Plus, practicing patience is a good way to grow. You can learn about yourself, become more aware of your moods and emotions, and be less reactive to the behaviors of guys you are hooking up with. You can't control them, only your own responses.

Tip #9:
YOU'RE FALLING FOR HIM—LET HIM KNOW.

You've met a couple of times, and you feel that you're falling for him. Honesty sets you free. I used to hide and lie about my feelings towards men I dated by omission. I pretended I was a casual lover and all I wanted was sex, which was usually true at the beginning —but that changed quickly, and I spent many lonely evenings crying into my pillow.

Throughout my first marriage, which lasted about three years, I never told my husband that I loved him. I was pretending to be cool, enjoying our open marriage (open marriage means that you can sleep with anyone you want and so can your partner). I acted like I didn't mind the enormous numbers of male and female lovers who crossed through our bedroom door—which wasn't completely false. The truth is that at first, I *did* enjoy the casualness of our relationship. He was my partner in crime and seduction, and we were a sexy and scandalous couple, hunting for new prey on a daily basis.

But then things changed.

I no longer liked the lifestyle we had. I wanted a change, but I didn't have the balls to tell him that I was suffering or that the situation was becoming unbearable for me. I was worried that I would scare him off, so I decided to hide my feelings from him forever. I was so unhappy, and the situation was so heavy, that I sought relief in drugs and alcohol. In the end, I lost him altogether—and he left me for someone else.

This story is dramatic, but if you feel that you're developing feelings for your casual lover, it's better to tell him the truth. Isn't it too early, you might ask? All the magazines are giving you advice to wait on the topic of serious dating or monogamy. I agree, but you have to be smart about how you ask. Don't text him about it. Meet up and tell him face to face, and express your wants and needs gently, without using demands or ultimatums. Be honest and say that although you expected to just have fun, he exceeded your expectations, and you are attracted to him! If you keep having such a great time with him, you might fall for him, and you aren't sure if that's what he would want.

While you talk, observe his body language and reaction. Is he nervous, not knowing where to look first, avoiding eye contact? Or is he smiling and obviously pleased to hear what you have to say? Does he share similar wishes about wanting a partner, or does he keep talking about casual sex and play parties?

Use your intuition, ladies. Men also have feelings, and they might like you more than you think. From my own experience, men also don't have a problem telling you they are not there yet, whether because of work or some other reason. The point here is that if you're on a completely different planet from him, the odds that you'll be hurt if you keep things going are very high. If you are falling for him and he just wants to play around, cut it off as soon as you can. Remember, the longer you stay around him, the worse it will be when you "break up."

Tip #10:
KEEP MULTIPLE LOVERS ON ROTATION

There is no "slutty, sluttier, and sluttiest"—you will be the same slut if you are fucking around with one guy or ten. I was slut-shamed early on as a teenager. My first sexual experience ended in disaster. The guy I considered my boyfriend at the time bragged about our sexual experience everywhere, and the whole town was pointing the finger at me. I was the sluttiest girl in town, just for having sex with one man. I was hurt, and since many men offered me their cock for my pleasure, I often took advantage of the offers and figured out this rotation rule pretty quickly.

As a sex and intimacy coach, many women have told me that they don't want to sleep with so many men because they would feel like sluts. I have the same response each time: why do women give up their own delight to be good girls? What's wrong with sluts? They are the best! They love their lives and cherish their sexuality. We live just once, and what others think is irrelevant.

But if you still give a fuck about other people's opinions, be a sly lover and have discreet fun. Nobody needs to know who performed acrobatics in your bedroom. A rule to remember is to pick guys from different circles, cities, and states. If you travel a lot, have lovers in different locations. Additionally, have a conversation with each of them and politely ask them to keep your affair private. It also helps to tell them that you'd like to keep it casual, as you're exploring your own sexuality. Men often love to hear this from a woman, as it ensures drama-free, no-strings-attached fun—and that's often all they can wish for.

In my personal journey, since I was already called "the Slut" from early on, I decided to take advantage of my new title. This rule came in handy when I was single and hooking up in New York City. What really protected my heart from being hurt was having multiple casual lovers on rotation. "Go hard or go home," said the shiny neon sign above my bed. When I got attached to Lover A, then Lover B fucked the attachment out of me. And then there was a C and occasionally also a D.

There were times when I liked one of them the most and missed him more, too. When that happened, I did a little exercise to bring myself back to being a cool cat. I wrote down the five most interesting and unique characteristics about each of my current flames. When I was with Lover A, I focused on the details I loved about him. When I was with Lover B, I did the same with him. That way I could focus on the best in the situation and stop thinking about the other guys. Ben was super fun, and we loved watching scientific videos after sex. I found it damn cute, something that Thomas would never do, but with him I would go to a Korean karaoke place and we would laugh our asses off. Thomas loved walks in nature and gave me a great back massage, but Ben's cock could hit my G-spot better. You see what I mean?

Multiple lovers keep you sane and give you the feeling of independence. It's like a war against oxytocin that makes you infatuated with someone you'd normally not give a damn about. Another advantage is that it helps you overcome jealousy. Do you have a feeling your hookup buddy is fucking around and is a player? Then guess what? You're the coach!

Once you have so many lovers that you get confused in remembering what you have done with whom, things get really funny. When this confusion happened to me, I couldn't remember: "Who was that guy trying to make me cum with a Polynesian orgasm technique—by blowing on my clit? Lord, was that ticklish!" It made me laugh hysterically. Nothing is better than being in a healthy spirit about your sex life.

Another advantage of having guys on rotation is that when one pisses you off, there are other ones left to treat you nicely. Good sex with one man can help you to get the other one you're obsessing about out of your system. Also, if you have a group of interesting lovers who keep you satisfied and entertained, it would be a shame to give them all up for that one guy after that one time. Unless he turns out to be Mr. Right and treats you like a queen—then you might reconsider. But my advice is to take your time.

Tip #11:
HIS REPLY WAS LAME—NO CALL TO ACTION

He is aloof.

"Hi handsome, how are you doing today?"

"Good!"

"Would you like to meet up this week?"

"Sorry, too busy."

You send him a cute/sexy pic and his reply is "nice" or "thanks."

He's being diplomatic, but he might as well tell you to stop bothering him, because that's exactly how these messages sound.

There is some wiggle room here, though. I understand that not every man is great with texting. Particularly, some men, especially those from generations older than the millennial generation, just don't text as much. It's simply not their cup of tea, and their messages might come across as boring or uninterested.

But follow your intuition, as I've said many times in this book. If he was texting you a lot before he got into your pants, and now, after a hookup, he doesn't seem to find a minute for a polite reply or suggest another rendezvous, the best choice here is to move on. My hunch is that this man will not play your game. He won't send you flirty, entertaining messages or be your occasional lover on your terms. He isn't interested in being either a friend with benefits or someone who is there to hug and comfort you when you need it. He is not interested in bringing this to another level. I know this might sound harsh and trust me, I know how sucky it feels! But you'll get over it! I want you to stay realistic and move on as soon as possible. Why? Because ambiguity hurts, and you don't want to waste more time thinking and fantasizing about this man.

Are you wondering what it's like in his head in these moments? I found out by asking men a key question: what would they do if the woman they slept with keeps reaching out to them and they don't want to see her again? Most of them said they would be polite and reply but wouldn't suggest another meeting. Eighty percent of these men would use the "I'm busy" excuse. So, in the majority of cases, if you get the "work has been so crazy lately" message, you know it's just a polite excuse that translates into "sorry, but I'm not interested."

Let's face it: nobody is too busy for sex! It's not only a fact that we already assumed, but those gentlemen confirmed it too. "Too busy for sex? Nobody is!" is what I frequently heard. Of course, sometimes men can be really busy, but if that's true, these men indicated they would say, "I'm busy tonight—how about next week, month, year?" Basically, they wouldn't let the chance to see you—and get laid again—slip through their hands.

When I asked them why they lie, they told me that they "don't want to hurt her feelings" and also wanted to leave the door open in case they are really bored and nobody else is around. When I called them on this as being unethical and immoral, they agreed but also admitted that sex is sex, and they will do, frankly, anything to get laid.

Despite this well-known truth, many women still live in the fantasy world of "what ifs," contemplating whether he is really busy, continuing to send free invitations to sex and suggestions to rendezvous.

For those who like to give second chances when he keeps saying he's busy with work, family, school, errands, etc., give yourself some tough love. You *know* that HE IS NOT THAT INTO YOU. So act like it! Also, understand that about 50 percent of men who say they are busy as an excuse the first time you contact them might not answer the next time you text them.

The rest of the gentlemen, another half, said that they would keep making excuses until the woman gives up and stops texting. Most of those men said that this strategy worked well for them in the past, and the woman will stop texting at some point.

To make it easier on you so you can close this chapter, ask yourself some important questions:

- What special element is he bringing to the equation?

- What can he offer you that you can't give yourself?

- What is so special about him that you want to spend your valuable energy and time to get him to like you and see you again?

Most likely, you will not know the answers to these questions and forget that he gave you an orgasm and made you feel good. You can express gratitude to your brain for producing all the feel-good and love hormones instead.

Sometimes craving a man is a way to fulfill the lack of something else in our life. You want what you don't have, and in this case it's him. Spare your energy, because trying to fulfill that lack of "him" is like playing the never-ending game of "lacking something." Once you get him, there will be another thing that you need to fulfill and will get attached to. Your personal fulfillment is the most important, so instead of chasing him, give yourself some self-love and do proper self-care. Others will follow.

Tip #12:
HE GHOSTED

It's an all-too-common scenario: Susan was disappointed, angry, and in disbelief after being ghosted (which means that one completely cuts off all contact and communication with you). The guy she'd met about a month ago—and had the hottest flirt with—disappeared after the second time they met for a playful night full of laugher and sex. She'd considered it a date and had hoped for the encounters to progress toward dating regularly, instead of just occasional sex. "After the second night we spent together he left my place in the morning, giving me a hug and a kiss, saying 'see you next time,'" she told me, clearly upset.

But this time, there was no follow-up text. Literally, no word from him. "After a couple of days, I texted to ask how he was doing, but I got no reply," she told me, "so I tried to call, but I got no answer. A couple of days later, I realized he'd blocked me from his Instagram account. I was going crazy! He could have simply said he wasn't into a relationship right now, and I wouldn't contact him again."

Of course, that didn't happen. Instead of a resolution, Susan felt bitter and uncomfortable, questioning what she had done wrong and why he had stopped liking her so suddenly.

As you can understand, ghosting can seriously mess with your head. But honestly, in regard to a person who does it, it's probably the best thing that could happen to you. Why? I consider it an ultimate asshole move. It's much worse than pulling the "I'm busy" card. Men who ghost these days are not worth losing a thought about, but when it happens, it's natural to think that something terrible happened to them. Was he run over by a bus? Did he have a death in his family? Most likely not, and he doesn't have the balls to be honest. Unless you're a crazy bitch who is stalking him at his office, texting him twenty times per day and calling his landline in the middle of the night, you deserve much better treatment.

In the interviews I conducted with men, only two out of fifty men said that when they don't want to see a woman again, they take the simplest solution and never reply. "Why would I reply?" one of them asked, smiling.

Sometimes you might wonder if he didn't see the text message or phone call. Sure, it happens. We can all miss notifications in our busy lives. In the case that he didn't block you from his social media accounts, as happened to Susan, you can calm your mind and give it one more shot. Simply ask, "Hope you're OK, since I haven't heard back." If there is no response to this, you know the answer.

I know it's natural to want to replay every moment with him and see where it went wrong but listen to me: don't torture yourself trying to figure out why he doesn't want to talk to you again. You could be rethinking possible scenarios for weeks. What if he was married or in a relationship? Was it something you did or didn't do in the bedroom? The possibilities are endless, and life is too short to speculate about them. And no—you do *not* need him to tell you he doesn't want to see you again and why. It's a form of closure we all crave to hear, sure, but we generally don't feel better after we do. He's not the one who should be giving you constructive criticism so you can learn for the next man. You are not a man-pleaser by profession. You are who you are, and if he didn't like you, it's his problem. Let him go.

I recognize this is easier said than done. Being ghosted might create a feeling of shame, and shame is one of the hardest things to let go of. It can make us feel that we fucked up or that we don't fit in. Then, in order to save our self-esteem, we will start blaming him, talking badly about him, and dwelling on all his flaws. By doing this, your psyche is just trying to repair its good self-image. It's normal, but be careful about how much time and energy you spend being surrounded by these negative feelings. My advice is rather to accept the rejection. Give yourself a big hug in front of the mirror, think about how much more free time you'll have to focus on more satisfying sexual partner-ships, and smile because it's clearly *his* big loss.

Tip #13:
YOU FOUND OUT HE IS FUCKING YOUR GIRLFRIEND. NOW WHAT?

This is really a crazy story that I heard from one of my closest friends. I wish I could disclose her name so she could confirm it's true, because it's totally unbelievable—but, obviously, I can't. Everything besides the names, though, is true in what I'm about to share. Get ready!

Melissa met Richard in a wine bar in Manhattan. He worked in finance and taught as a professor at a prestigious university. They had a fun conversation, and he smelled so good—like aromatic oils of scents she had never smelled before. She was intrigued. After a couple of dates, he invited her to his chic downtown apartment. After the dinner he had cooked, he offered her a massage. He kept bragging about his outstanding massage skills until she gave in and found herself topless, lying on the fur on his sofa. He rubbed oil onto her back, spent about five minutes around her shoulders, and quickly made his way to her breasts.

It didn't take long before they moved to his bedroom to play. But then Melissa felt like she was in a *zoo*. Richard made weird animal sounds. His long, curly hair was all over her face and in her mouth, and he squeaked loudly, in a high-pitched voice, into her ear while fucking her, making the weirdest melodramatic faces. "I'm so good, do you feel my cock? Am I a great lover? Tell me, you're freaking out, aren't you?" he kept repeating. Feeling his drool on her ear and neck was the last straw, and she pretended to come just to get it over with.

What a Zoolander! Melissa told herself when leaving his house.

They met up a couple more times afterward, as Melissa wanted to give him a second chance. All he could talk about were his incredible sex skills, asking her if she liked the orgasm and wanted more. Richard tried everything possible to impress Melissa. He kept texting her, inviting her over for more "tantric sex," and telling her he was falling for her. She liked him and wondered how she could train him to be a better lover.

When her girlfriend Janette came to visit from Chicago, Melissa told her all about him, hoping Janette could provide her with some advice. Janette was super happy that her friend had met a cool guy, and she wanted to see his picture. After Melissa revealed a photo of them cuddled up in his bedsheets, Janette froze. "Oh gosh, Melissa—I'm fucking him too! In fact, he offered to let me stay at his house tomorrow night, so I saved money on a hotel. We met at a conference in Austin!"

Melissa looked at her friend in shock. They were in the same crowd of people, but what were the odds they would be hooking up with the same man? Jealousy mixed with disappointment—and was followed by laughter. They began comparing notes. He had been sending them the same pictures and telling them the same things. Nothing creative or unique! Neither was upset with him, though. It was only casual sex, and nobody was claiming to be monogamous.

"Look, Janette, go and stay with him tomorrow," Melissa said. "I won't say anything, but I can't see him again. I honestly lost my appetite—it's too close to home. Also, Ashley is coming from Florida and staying with me, and I'll be hanging out with her all afternoon."

"Oh, I love Ashley! Haven't seen her in a while. Let's all have some wine, and then I'll decide if I'll see him or not," suggested Janette.

The next afternoon, they met in the lobby of Janette's hotel. Over glasses of wine, Ashley shared a story about a young man she had hooked up with a couple of times in the past and was supposed to see the following night. They had met at a conference in Boston about a year earlier. She kept describing him, and at some point, Janette and Melissa looked at each other. "Is his name Richard?" they asked in unison.

Ashley looked at them like a deer in the headlights. It was the same guy! They couldn't believe it and kept marveling at the ridiculousness of the situation. "He's acting like such a Zoolander, so ridiculous!" Melissa yelled, and they all burst out laughing.

The messages he was sending them were all the same, the dick pics were all the same, and he literally had them lined up one night after the other to come to his house. They compared the sex details and came up with a great idea: to text him and invite him to join them for wine. "Let's play with the player," said Janette. "I'm supposed to see him tonight, so I can suggest the meeting. To see all of us will be a great surprise!"

And so they did. "Richard will be here in five minutes!" said Janette, and Ashley and Melissa ran to hide in the bathroom of a local bar. Upon his arrival, he sat next to Janette, and soon after, the girls showed up by the table. His jaw dropped, and he stared at them in disbelief. "Oh, hi, Ashley, what are you doing here?" he asked. "Oh, Melissa, hi, I didn't know you guys were friends. Wow, WTF! Small world. I have no words!" he kept bumbling.

"You and no words, Richard? Never!" laughed Ashley.

The whole situation is unbelievable, but it's a real story. He felt uncomfortable beyond belief and lost his three lovers in one day. None of the ladies wanted to see him again—and not because he had many lovers. We live in a world where having more than one lover is OK, but not many want to see the other affairs right in front of their faces. It takes the mystery away and ruins the fantasy. I've been in situations where I had casual lovers for years, and they were so unsophisticated about their other affairs that I lost interest. To assume you're not the only one a man is sleeping with is one thing, but discovering his other lovers—especially when they're your friends—is a deal-breaker for many women.

We all want fantasy and not reality. Sometimes I found used condoms in my lover's trash can. Another time I found used panties in another guy's bed while we were playing. These are just unsexy moments that ruin the erotic vibe. So, guys (and ladies, too)—play around, but do your research beforehand. Perhaps checking social media and seeing if your lovers know each other wouldn't hurt, right?

The question remains: what do you do when you learn that your hookup is fucking your best friend? If he lied to you, punish him. Maybe you and your friend can create an embarrassing situation you will lure him into—one he won't forget. Make sure you're safe, as men don't always react well to being embarrassed by women. If he didn't lie, you can decide if you still want to see him, knowing he's fucking your BFF. After all, sharing is sometimes caring. And, depending on your naughtiness and jealousy level, you can plan a hot ménage à trois.[7] For some, the more, the merrier!

---

[7] A sexual encounter involving three people; a threesome.

Tip #14:
DO NOT TAKE THINGS PERSONALLY— EVER!

Most of the time when people critique us, it's not really about us—it's about them. Their frustrations. Their shortcomings. Their unfulfilled needs.

But even though we know this to be true, remembering it when we are hurt is a different story—just like this one I dealt with recently from a client.

When Samantha received a message from James that he wasn't into a relationship right now and would stop seeing her, she was surprised. "He called me clingy and said that he feels I'm looking for more commitment than he can offer me! I only saw him three or four times, and on each date, we had a stellar time! When we were apart, I kept communicating with him daily, but only one or two sweet and sexy messages to keep the anticipation for our next date going," she said. "I also asked when we should meet again, as I like to plan and look forward to another rendezvous. I'd like to give myself fully into that moment and want to be prepared for the evening of sex. You know what I mean. Mani, pedi, sexy outfit. It's a big part of the fun! I guess that wasn't what he was looking for. Maybe I was texting too much and overwhelmed him? What do you think, Lia?"

She kept asking me these questions in our coaching session, and I could tell that his words of blame had gotten deep under her skin. "Once, he texted in the morning that he had a meeting close to my house and asked if he could stop by for an afternoon delight. He knew I worked from home. I said yes, but I felt like a booty call!" Samantha said with disappointment. "And then last week, I was walking my dog in the park and spotted him making out with another woman on a park bench! He was holding her hand, looking into her eyes, playing with her hair. That woman laughed back at him flirtatiously, and they started French kissing. I was standing in the grass behind them waiting for my dog to do his thing and then walked away as fast as I could. They seemed so in love with each other! I was jealous and furious! She was blonder and skinnier than me! Wearing a beautiful coat that I probably can't even afford." I had to stop Samantha from hurting herself with more words.

When someone treats us unkindly or without respect, we tend to take things personally and begin wondering about our body, beauty, and behavior. This is emotionally draining. It is a constant reevaluation of our self-esteem. The fact that he ghosted, told us we are "not for him," or—even worse—criticized us for something we did while together, can start a lengthy process of overthinking and not being able to let go.

Here's what to remember: when he is honest, appreciate his words as clear facts and move on with your sexy ass. When he criticizes you in order to create a false sense that his departure is your fault, do not buy into it. Criticizing or blaming you for anything is a sign that he can't take responsibility for his own actions, and it's a sign of emotional immaturity. Better that he's gone, right? Because that's not what you need in a potential partner.

Taking things personally can result in you questioning your strengths and qualities, such as your intelligence ("does he think I'm not too smart?"), humor ("maybe the jokes I was making yesterday were too silly"), beauty ("I think I'm too skinny/too fat for him"; "maybe he likes smaller/bigger boobs"). This can get ridiculous.

I've met women who were questioning their age, education, apartment décor, or even lack of foreign language skills! When I see this happening, I just want to shout, "STOP" at them and interrupt this harmful thought process.

No more comparing. Understand that his leaving is not about you. Not only that, but know that he is not worth driving yourself crazy thinking this way! Not taking things personally gives you more control over your emotions and protects you from feeling too crushed after a negative hookup experience.

Most importantly, know your worth and who you are. In a survey I conducted in the summer of 2019 for my final thesis at Columbia University, I asked 250 individuals about the factors that give them power in a relationship. The most important factor was self-esteem. If you are self-confident and know your value, nobody can convince you otherwise. Even if he never reaches out to you again, it's because you're most likely "overqualified" and he got scared. You are powerful enough to change your thoughts and be on top of things, so let an experience like this empower you to feel better and sexier rather than drag you down into anger, bitterness, and low self-esteem.

Tip #15:
HOW TO GET RID OF YOUR ADICKTION

D o you feel empty when he is not inside of you? Did he make you feel good with his tongue, penis, or hands—or all of the above—and now you can't stop thinking of him? If he's on your mind around your parents, in the office, gym, shower, and even when meditating, the answer is: you are addicted! But no worries—this is totally natural. Research shows that you can fall in love with someone in a fifth of a second![8] The orgasm and sexual connection with this beau shot your oxytocin levels through the roof. Because oxytocin is a euphoria-inducing chemical that makes you feel in love, the strong attachment after a short hookup is backed up by science. In addition, attraction and romantic love may activate our brain's opioid system, which is involved in pleasure. This combination can make us literally addicted to the feelings and hormones of love in the same way as cocaine. So, guess what, ladies—the addiction is real!

---

[8] Stephanie Ortigue, Francesco Bianchi-Demicheli, Nisa Patel, Chris Frum, and James W. Lewis, "Neuroimaging of Love: FMRI Meta-Analysis Evidence toward New Perspectives in Sexual Medicine," *The Journal of Sexual Medicine* 7, no. 11 (November 2010): 3541–52, https://doi.org/10.1111/j.1743-6109.2010.01999.x.

If you are still hooking up with him, you will be getting your dose of dick on a regular basis, which will most likely keep you an addict. In that case, enjoy it as much as you can without turning into a total zombie, unable to focus on anything else in your life. If you are not hooking up with him anymore and you're going through a tough withdrawal, don't worry. You will get over it soon. I wish I could provide you an exact number of days that you will be obsessing, but unfortunately, there is no way to know. Every situation is unique.

For me personally, when I was totally addicted, I needed about two weeks to let go of the attachment. The length of your addiction also depends on how often and how much you were hooking up with this particular guy. Let's say that if you were hooking up for a month, you should be fine in a couple of weeks. If it's half a year, you will probably need three months to recover. Heads up—the more days that pass by from the last time you saw him, the less you're going to miss him!

If you're feeling the withdrawal from your addicktion, there is no point in fighting it. Accept it and acknowledge that it shall soon pass, and you'll be free as a bird. In the meantime, on difficult days, do things for yourself. Take a walk, meditate, and masturbate watching porn or thinking of someone else. Do not go back into thinking about your experiences with him or imagining his dick.

And by all means, please avoid going to the sex shop, buying yourself a same-sized dildo, and naming it after him. That could make you crave his dick even more, and that's not what you want right now.

Every time the thought of his penis arrives, think of something else immediately! Perhaps turn your thoughts to ice cream, hot coffee, or a vacation you're about to take. Tell yourself strictly: *stop, stop, stop*! Count colors you are seeing around you or count from one hundred to one backward in increments of seven. Keep changing your thoughts of him until you stop thinking of him altogether. Retrain your brain and reclaim your a*dick*tion-free life!

Tip #16:
NO BLAME

Ever had a hookup not go as planned—so much so that you wished you'd stayed home? It happened to Jane. She'd met Matt on Tinder and, due to their busy schedules, they messaged online for many months before an actual date took place. Matt was an excellent writer. He sent Jane sexy poems, ideas for dates, and flattering messages that turned her on incredibly. He even sent her flowers one day. The anticipation was real, and she was excited to have met a great guy.

The big night arrived. Jane and Matt met in a chic cocktail bar. Soon after he arrived, Jane felt he was not as fun as he was in his messages. He looked kind of dorky, and his clothing lacked a sense of style. Jane had a fantasy of a chic, well-dressed Romeo, and although she had seen his pictures, he was not as she expected him to be. He was clumsy and spilled a cocktail on her new dress. When they walked toward the elevators, leaving the bar, he stepped on her foot.

Already annoyed, Jane wanted to just call it a day and go home in huge disappointment, but they planned to go to his place. She didn't want to change the agenda. He was so dorky and clumsy, though, and she had a hunch he wouldn't be a good lover. Quite frankly, she wasn't even into him anymore.

Yet there she was, in his bedroom in a small studio in Brooklyn, styled with sports caps and pennants of sports teams. How sexy!

"Would you like to have a beer?" he asked. She nodded and looked around his little place. It was clean, at least. When he came closer to her and squeezed himself next to her on the sofa, he was shaking and totally nervous. She just wanted to have this over and to go home, so they fucked. As she expected, it was super boring, and he was a clumsy lover. "Sweet guy, but…" she thought the next day, deconstructing this date. "Never again—I should have known better, stupid me!"

If your hookup doesn't go as planned, it's better to stay away from assigning blame to yourself or your date. Blame is similar to victimization; it's an unhealthy reaction that doesn't serve any useful purpose. There are two sides of the spectrum in the blame game. On one side, there are people who will find someone or something to put the blame on about pretty much everything, not only in dating or sex. On the other side, there are some people who will blame themselves for everything, even if they have nothing to do with the poor outcome. What side of the spectrum are you on? Read further and I'll explain how this behavior could have harmful effects on your life in the long run.

Do you hear yourself saying, "He deceived me!"? I would never go out with him otherwise!" or "He got me so drunk that I vomited all over him!" or "He forgot to get the vegan, latex-free, and cruelty-free condoms from our local organic store, and we had to stop in the best moment! How dare he?"

Why do we blame others for things when *we had the same amount of control over the outcome?*

First of all, blaming others is a great defense mechanism and helps to preserve our self-esteem. It's harder to admit that we saw the red flags, kind of expected this might happen, and still didn't take precautionary steps to avoid the potential negative outcome. Blaming others protects our ego, as it's easier to blame someone else for an unfortunate situation than to take accountability for our own actions.

Do you say, "I'm so sorry" obnoxiously often, or do you have friends like that? Are you wondering why they blame themselves all the time? The reasons vary, but sometimes they are looking for reassurance from people because they don't feel they're enough. Taking on guilt for something that is obviously not their fault will make others say, "Don't worry, it's not your fault," which is perhaps what they need to hear in order to feel better about themselves. There are also individuals who hate conflict and will do anything to avoid it—even if that's taking the blame themselves before someone else can do it.

You might have a tendency toward *internal attributions for failure,* where you can see yourself as foolish, incompetent, thoughtless, or other "fun" descriptors you give yourself or believe in because your parents, friends, and others called you those things. To be seen as such will help you easily explain future failures and understand "why things always keep happening to you again." Women tend to attribute their failures to internal factors much more than men. Dear ladies, it's time to stop with this guilt. Stop saying you're sorry for too many things. "Sorry I had sex with you, and it was bad" has no place in my book.

You must find the right balance between owning things and asking others for improvement. Stay out of the pattern of playing the blame game. The more you play it, the more you might lose.

Tip #17:
BELIEVE WHATEVER YOU WANT TO BELIEVE

In my work with women, I see a common theme: your relationship happiness and dating life can be totally ruled by your limiting beliefs, if you're not careful. Limiting beliefs are thoughts that hold us back in some ways, often regarding our self-identities and ourselves.

How does this play out in real life? Take a look: I recently hosted a workshop for women. Some of the women were married and some were single, and they seemed to have similar issues around dating. Some of them felt they had too much power and became bored and frustrated in a relationship with a partner who wasn't assertive enough. Some of them felt they let the man they were dating take too much control and ended up feeling disempowered, unable to take their power back. I listened closely to their stories:

"Once he knew he had control over me and that I was in love with him, he began telling me what to do. I literally felt like his submissive and couldn't resist his wishes. I've always had issues in saying no to people. In the end he left me for another woman anyways. Who would want to be with such a lap dog?" said Charlotte.

"And I have a completely different problem," said Isabella. "My husband isn't assertive enough, and I'm so annoyed by him always saying yes to me. Our relationship doesn't work—I'm too dominant for him."

Another lady, Kate, went on to tell her story: "All guys leave me after a couple of dates. I'm not assertive enough, and the last guy I was seeing left me for another woman because I didn't make a clear move and never told him about my feelings. It's a shame—I really liked him."

Listening to all their stories, I saw the limiting beliefs right away. Where do these come from, you might ask? We gather them from our experiences in personal and professional settings—from interactions with family, friends, and partners. Sometimes those are deeply rooted and come from our family system and childhood. Here are some examples:

- "I'm too powerful, and all men are scared of me!"

- "Men think I'm a submissive little play toy."

- "No man loves me!"

- "There are no good guys out there!"

- "I'm too horny—I can never wait."

- "I will never find a boyfriend."

- "I can't live without him."

- "I can't be monogamous/polyamorous."

- "All men cheat and fuck around."

- "I always get attached/hurt after a hookup."

At the end of the workshop, curious to find what they believed was the problem in their respective relationships, I decided to have a quick chat with each of the women separately. Listening to them, I realized that the limiting beliefs they carried within themselves became their personal mantras that directly disabled them from growth and change. They couldn't see, let alone improve upon, the unhealthy patterns that no longer suited them.

These women aren't rare in this. Many of us do the same thing! We are masters in creating limiting beliefs—and not only around our dating lives.

When you're going on a date with this kind of attitude, you're already scripting the outcome, so why even bother to go on a date in the first place? Why would you make all that effort just to be with a guy who's going to cheat and fuck around anyway? Why would you want to go for dinner and have sex with a man who will be scared of you and never call you again, as all of them did in the past? You see what I mean?

Now is the time to change the way you think about yourself, men, and love in general. I agree that undoing these constraining stories that were part of your life and identity for many years can be hard, yet it's an achievable task. First, it's important to recognize limiting beliefs. Then you must reframe the sentences you're using that no longer suit you, such as "I'm too powerful and all men are scared of me." You must rewire your brain with positive affirmations. Instead, imagine a new reality that you'd like to live in, and talk about it— loudly, if necessary.

The issue is that when living through your limiting beliefs, you can subconsciously act in a way that comes across as dominant in an unsexy way. Unless you want to be a dominatrix and have a submissive man, you need to change this way of thinking. Look for opportunities to surrender control, take a softer approach, and leave room for him to initiate.

Your visualizations and the stories you're telling yourself have enormous power. As Dr. Dispenza says, you will create a reality based on your thoughts. Once you change your thoughts, you will change your reality.

Tip #18:
GRATITUDE AMPLIFIES

Life is all about experiences, and nothing—that's right, nothing—lasts forever. As humans, though, we tend to hold on to things and people so tightly that we can't have gratitude and focus for the present moment.

This is a hard lesson, but one my client Cathy learned beautifully.

"I will remember and cherish these moments forever. No matter what comes," said Damon, leaving Cathy's hotel room following their afternoon tryst. He had escaped from a conference, and she took off from work. Cathy and Damon only hooked up a couple of times. It was a short affair, but their sexual connection was intense, definitely sex to remember. She enjoyed his company very much and loved talking to him. Prior to their hookup, they'd had coffee dates where they could talk for hours. Damon was a smart and sophisticated man with a great sense of humor.

You may be thinking: He sounds great! What's the issue? It's logistical: Damon was in the midst of moving to another country due to his work, and neither of them knew if they would see each other again.

"It sucks to meet a great lover in the time when he's moving to another continent," said Cathy with sadness as she shared her experience with me over coffee in Manhattan. "As bittersweet as it might sound, it is a beautiful story that provides a lot of learning, and I'm forever grateful I could experience this connection. I enjoyed every minute of it fully. I have never paid so much attention to every detail with one man!"

Cathy explained she'd dedicated herself to being present the entire time. Instead of worrying about her hair, outfit, and performance, she became completely focused on the moment. She told me it was like the world around didn't exist. Because she didn't—and wouldn't—know, Cathy wasn't obsessing over when she'd see Damon again. She also wasn't worried about being too naughty.

"I was being the wild me. I kept looking into his eyes, carefully observing his face, body, skin. I kissed his lips and wanted to absorb as many little memories as I could from that, perhaps our last afternoon," she shared. "I was simply grateful for being there at that moment."

As I listened to her, I wondered, why don't we live our whole lives like this? Absorbing the beauty of the moment, full of gratitude, not worrying about tomorrow?

Imagine you're meeting a friend for lunch. You have a conversation that you pay attention to a bit. Perhaps you both judge one another's hairstyle or outfit inwardly while you outwardly share some news about your lives. Then you look around the place, checking your phone every once in a while, until it's time to say goodbye. You're most likely taking for granted that you'll see them again, so the idea to soak in every little detail of the interaction isn't even in your head. "See you next week, next month, in LA, in Paris"—who knows what plans you made, but there's no guarantee! Be grateful to see your friend and cherish the moments you got to spend together.

The same is applicable with your hookup. Don't obsess over whether you'll see him again and think about what's next while you're with him. Live in the now, as best you can, and be grateful for that! Communicate, share, and absorb. Instead of being worried about your performance and the extra two pounds that nobody besides you cares about, pay attention to him and the words he is saying. Have a meaningful conversation. Learn about him and from him.

After the hookup, even if you'll never see him again, appreciate the connection and experience you had with this person. Express gratitude for the moments and memories, the kisses, laughter, sensual moments, and sex in general without greed and neediness. The more you're grateful for the experience, the more you'll get from the Universe.

Tip #19:
MANAGING YOUR EXPECTATIONS

Expectations are a great route to disappointment. The more you expect, the more you'll get hurt. This goes for many expectations in our lives, but especially for hookups.

Think about it: you don't know the guy at all, and you are basically expecting magic from someone who doesn't know you either. Still, sadly, most of us have expectations around casual sex! Research[9] has shown that women and men both have expectations, but their ideal outcomes differ. Among women, 43 percent indicated that a romantic relationship is the ideal outcome, followed by friendship at 24 percent, and then further hookups, wished for by only 17 percent of women. For men, 32 percent would ideally have an ongoing sexual relationship with the woman they hooked up with, 29 percent a romantic relationship, and 24 percent a friendship.

This means that one in three men you hook up with would be interested in a relationship with you. And since men will never say no to sex, the women who want to have an ongoing, NSA (no strings attached) relationship will also find their satisfaction. As this research shows, only 15 percent of men are not interested in having more contact with the women they hook up with. Therefore, statistically speaking, there's a five-times-higher chance that you'll see this guy

---

[9] Weitbrecht and Whitton, "Expected, Ideal, and Actual Relational Outcomes of Emerging Adults' 'Hook Ups,'" 902–16.

again than that you won't. So, manage your expectations and keep it cool. The best way is to have zero outside-the-bed expectations when it comes to casual lovers. You have no idea who he is or his real reason for hooking up.

How can you manage your expectations, though? First, don't expect others to behave the way you would. Many of us make the mistake of comparing ourselves to others. Then we judge other people's actions and behaviors because they are different from ours. When it comes to your hookup, you don't want to be naïve and expect him to be nice and reach out to you the same way you would. There is no guarantee, as we all have different communication and dating styles. Set your most important expectations straight, know what makes you happy, and once you have known him longer or seen him for more dates, communicate your wishes. If he fulfills them, great. If not, say goodbye.

Finally, the only behavior I expect from everyone is kindness. It's the minimum that humans can give to each other.

Tip #20:
DESIRE IS NOT WHAT IT SEEMS

Men love challenges—don't forget that. Of course, he can desire you too, but often the desire for challenge is masked behind desire for someone, and the most difficult thing is telling the difference. He can be a seducer, and you might be his target. He plays the seduction game with you, and once you give in too fast, you will lose your power and be at his mercy. Please keep in mind that he might not even desire you as a person, and you may be merely another challenge for him. In that case, his interest will wane right after you have sex.

A proper game of seduction takes time; you might not want to spend that time and effort on this particular man, and that's OK. Or you might not be in the mood to have your seducer luring you into his trap, and you only want quick sexual pleasure. In that case, go for it. Be warned, though: I've seen this happen many times in my life and the lives of many other women, and our hormones can go crazy. Though our intentions may have been to have only casual sex, things can turn otherwise.

For ladies who wish to be seduced, taken on a journey by a "Casanova," and thrive on the feeling of being a man's desire, remember that he might desire challenge more than he desires you. Skilled seducers can get under your skin way too deep, so before you hook up, think about this man and his goal. If he's worth your interest, let him play for longer. Make it difficult for him and enjoy the play of seduction he has prepared for you.

If you gave in too fast (because of your insatiable craving for sex and fear that he'd stop), now that he's gone, don't let this experience make you bitter. Take it as an opportunity to get to know yourself better and observe how this made you feel. Do you feel comfortable getting your pleasure in return for his ignorance, or do you wish for him to be around more and give you some attention? Do you experience negative feelings that last longer than the whole encounter and seduction? Then reconsider your next hookup, because casual sex is probably not for you, and you're looking for a different and longer-lasting scenario.

When you feel like a target of his desire for challenge, you can do two things: politely tell him you're not interested, as this game is uncomfortable for you—or, as I've already mentioned above, if you want to play, make it really difficult for him. Be less approachable in your responses. When he's pulling away, be sweet. When he thinks he has you, push him away and be aloof or cold. Confuse him. Maybe you'll be the one who seduces him at the end, and he might fall for you. Or perhaps he'll move on to another target, but at least you can enjoy a fun game and prepare a lot of obstacles on his way into your pants.

Tip #21:
FIGURE OUT WHAT YOU ARE ACTUALLY CRAVING

Are you sure you're craving the man you just hooked up with, or is it something else you're missing in your life? Some women want to fulfill their needs for intimacy, attention, and closeness through sex, and I do not recommend taking this route. Once the sex is over, you can feel empty and sad because the short sexual act only provided a touch of closeness and intimacy—one that lasted only as long as he did.

The antidote to this reaction is to deconstruct the origin of your cravings in the first place. Is there anything so special about him that you can't find in other men or your friends? You might be infatuated and say he is so smart, tall, funny, etc. But be real! Quite frankly, many other men are, too. Plus, it's impossible to know him after only the couple of times you've met him. It takes longer to discover the real qualities in people, so you're most likely craving him because he fucked your brains out.

How do you find out if you're subconsciously using him as a tool to satisfy your other needs? Take him completely out of the equation and see if you can find a pattern in your behavior with other men in the past. What if you're just trying to fulfill the needy little girl who is still ruling your adult world?

This can be difficult to fully let soak in, so here's an example from my own life. For many years, I longed to be around older men. Ever since I was a teenager, my boyfriends were fifteen, twenty, or thirty years older than me. I felt safe around them and enjoyed the attention and advice they gave me. I needed them, and the idea of not having these older men in my life freaked me out.

Then, in my mid-thirties, I realized I had a daddy complex. Through coaching and therapy, I analyzed my childhood and remembered how much I missed my dad as a little girl. My dad worked thousands of miles away from home, traveling to Russia, France, and other countries. He came home to my mom and me only every two weeks. I still remember how much I looked forward to seeing him and how sad and anxious I was when he was leaving. I often woke up at 4 a.m. when he arrived just to give him a hug. Due to the lack of his presence, I longed for him and his attention. I tried everything under the sun to get more of his attention, which was difficult due to his busy work schedule.

This need projected itself into my adult love life. Beginning when I was sixteen, I preferred to be around much older men. I needed to date a powerful male figure who also gave me immense attention. I wasn't interested in dating younger men at all. They just didn't do it for me.

At some point, I didn't care what function an older man had in my life. He could be my friend, lover, or boyfriend. He always needed me, too, as someone to take care of—and not necessarily financially. Often, this was only mentally, and their reward was acknowledgment and respect—something they had been lacking since childhood and didn't get from their parents or, often, wives.

I was stuck in this pattern for almost two decades, until I realized that I wanted to change and didn't need a daddy. Getting unstuck was difficult, and I sought professional help from coaches and psychotherapists who helped me to realize that I'm smart, powerful, and don't need anyone in my life in order to feel good about myself and trust my decisions.

I'm glad I did the work and began to feel excited about dating younger, more marriage- and family-eligible men. I broke the unhealthy cycle in my early thirties. I still believe I wouldn't mind dating an older man if the situation were right. After all, age is just a number, and I find older men just as sexy as younger men. For me, though, that relationship would have to be based on attraction, good sex, and healthy power dynamics—not a daddy-daughter dependence pattern.

To come to your own happy ending, discover what it is you're craving. Then, acknowledge where it is coming from and know that you, too, are a powerful and strong woman who can give yourself all the love and appreciation you need. You are enough! Meditate and masturbate on it.

Tip #22:
PLAY WITH POWER

Sex is not just for pleasure and making babies. There are many other functions of this encounter. Thousands of years ago, power was gained through physical strength and violence in fights or wars. Women had no chance to succeed because of their physiological features and struggled under this arrangement. But as we all know, men lose their minds and often think irrationally when they want pussy.

The biggest weakness of men is ultimately their unappeasable desire for sex. That means women can use this male weakness to their advantage. I was never an advocate of waiting too long for the first time, as you know by now. But unfortunately, often when we give a man sex before he's emotionally invested, we also lose our power. That means there's a huge chance that he will start looking elsewhere. Before you give away your power, make sure it is something you want to risk.

It's like gambling in a casino. If you like the adrenaline of the game and you don't care about losing the money, go for it. But if you can be psychologically harmed, play with him a bit and keep the power in your hands. Find the perfect balance of wit, intelligence, and sexiness. Seduce his mind and brain. Be a fun friend—offer him something that he can't do with anyone else. Have a meaningful conversation about an important topic and throw a bit of flirting and seduction into the mix.

If you drag him to your house, you tease him madly, you both undress, and then, when he's hard, hot, and horny for you, you interrupt the game—it's a terrible way of doing it. He might feel tricked, and you can end up in an argument. If you offer him a hand job or a blowjob instead, it has the same effect as sex. Once he has an orgasm, he's got what he wanted and might never reach out to see you again. Plus, he can think of you as being unfair for teasing him and not letting him sleep with you. My suggestion is to leave the petting and nudity for another time and make him crave you and want to see you more. This is a game that requires patience and some strategizing, so you had better make sure he's worth it.

Again, if you only want a quick lay, disregard my advice in this matter and use his cock for your pleasure.

Once I met a super-sexy man in Miami. He was in his late twenties, played sports, and had an incredibly ripped body and olive skin. On top of that, he was smart, witty, and had money. The full package, you might think. We became friends, and I have to admit I got wet just being around him. His slightly arrogant nature and his playing it cool made him even more attractive. He played the hard-to-get game, and he did it really well.

I was going crazy, and I wanted to have sex with him. One day we got super drunk and, with his other guy friend, ended up in his condo in South Beach. His place was huge, with incredible views. We were drinking shots of tequila, smoking hookah on the balcony, and watching the lights of the Miami skyline. Then he began talking about his last prey. Typical dude-talk. But the conversation got indiscreet, and he began showing his friend nude pictures of women he'd had sex with in recent weeks. He laughed about how easy they were to get. I felt uncomfortable, as I found it lame and unfair to the women. "And I got another Polaroid on my string!" he said, and his friend asked, "How many do you have already?"

"Over two hundred! Dude, I'm losing track—should we count?" he replied.

"Yeah, let's go," answered his friend, and they both left the balcony and headed toward one of his rooms. I followed them, as I was very curious what "Polaroid on the string" meant. He opened the door of a room that looked like his office and switched the light on. At the end of the room, there was a long string attached from the right to the left wall, covered with Polaroid pictures of naked women. The small pictures were hanging on the string with clothespins. I couldn't believe it! There were hundreds!

"Incredible! Cheers, dude!" said his friend, and they clinked their glasses and drank another shot of tequila. At some point, the host looked at me. My facial expression was a mixture of disgust, shock, and interest in his perversion. I have to say my desire to sleep with this man was immediately gone, and every time I had a hookup with an obvious player, I wondered what number on the Polaroid string I would be.

The same rule applies here too. Only invest as much in the game as you're ready to lose. If he's a player and you're a coach, have fun and collect your own Polaroids! If you are looking for something deeper, be careful and take it slowly.

If he really played you and now you have lost power and are feeling miserable, imagine how much this low-self-esteem brat would suffer without your help. You helped him to feel like himself again, and you got some karma points there. Do yourself a favor and never call him again. If he needs to boost his ego by getting into your pants, then by calling him you'll double down on his pleasure and increase his self-esteem. He might even think that his performance was so irresistible that you can't live without it!

It's sad, but this dynamic is still so prevalent in our society that some men don't realize that women can be crushed after such arrogant experiences. Although I'm not here to try to change men, I would like to make them more aware. Man or woman, the only person that can change your approach to casual sex and sex in general is *you*.

Tip #23:
NO SHAME OR GUILT

These days, many women feel empowered to ask for pleasure, but then something can feel not quite right after we do. That's what happened to one Joanna, who shared this story:

"One night I was extremely turned on by the fantasy of having sex with Andy. I was imagining the last time I saw him, remembering his tall, lean frame and his musky smell—so sexy and sensual. I could still hear his calm, deep voice that was so pleasant to listen to, and I had to remind myself to pay attention to his words instead of being drawn into his deep blue eyes. I only knew Andy professionally. He worked in the same building in New York as I did, thankfully on a different floor. We met in a cafeteria near our office on our lunch break. After some initial small talk, we engaged in an interesting conversation that continued until we got into the elevator to go back to work. As he was leaving, he handed me his business card, saying, 'Why don't you reach out and we can continue the conversation?' I agreed and thought that perhaps we could grab another lunch or coffee at some point.

"But you know how things turn out when you're single and a cold night in New York City approaches. One of these lonely evenings, I found his card and texted to ask if we could meet up the next day for coffee. After the text went out, before I even got a reply, I got a strange feeling in my stomach. I was ashamed and felt bad that I had even texted him. *What is he going to think when I'm texting him at 9 p. m.? He must believe that I'm lonely and horny. What if…* blah, blah, blah. My brain went on until late at night, and his reply came late as well.

"The next morning, with mixed feelings, I changed my outfit three times and rushed out of my apartment to meet him. There he was, sitting on the corner, wearing a black coat and white-and-blue striped shirt and a tie. He was a clean-cut man, with precise features and thick, short brown hair. 'Good morning, you look very elegant today,' he said, giving me a compliment on my maybe 'too sexy for work' beige sweater dress and high-heeled boots. He immediately stood up to pull out the chair for me.

"Our conversation was even more pleasant than the first time, and we walked back to the office together. In the elevator, I was the one who became greedy for more. I'd been single for over two years, and other than some casual one-night stands, I had no steady lover. 'Mornings are very rushed for me—how about we have dinner next time,' I said and looked at him with a seductive smile. He just smiled back. 'Sure, next week?'

"I agreed and moved on with my day. Although I was very excited to see him again, that other voice in my head didn't stop bugging me for the whole week. *You shouldn't be the one suggesting a rendezvous.* 'Oh, come on,' I said to myself, 'women are empowered. We can do it too.' Even so, I heard another voice. *You ruined the thrill of seduction for him*, said the voice in my head again, and I felt ashamed.

"The whole week, I focused my energy on the night we were supposed to meet. Everything went well. No cancellations, no delays! The dinner was in a beautiful, sultrily lit restaurant not too far from his place. We had wine, and at some point, he invited me to his house. I didn't say no to that because I was absolutely sure I wanted to have sex with him.

"The sex was great, as it usually is when you have two or three drinks. It was wild. It was loud. He came. I think I did, too. Or perhaps I didn't, but I had fun. He even went down on me for a brief minute. Because it was a Thursday night and because I barely knew his last name, I decided to go home after a couple of pleasurable rounds.

"The next morning, I woke up with a horrible hangover, late for work, with JBF hair. As I showered, I felt mortified about what I had done. *I'm a slut. He works in the same building. How will I act if I see him?*

What will I say? I must quit that job. I need to relocate. Words of hysteria went through my head. I was plainly ashamed, confused, and felt guilty that I had gone too far. I was feeling bad that I had sex with a man I barely knew, and that I had initiated it. I was worried about what would come next! I totally regretted it, even though I had a pleasant experience!"

Joanna's story, sadly, didn't have a happy ending. The next morning Andy reached out and exchanged some messages with her, but she gave only one-word replies. When they ran into each other in the elevator, Joanna, full of shame, just acted awkwardly. She was so sure that he would not want to see her again, because he looked like a proper man and she saw herself as a slut, that her weirdness pushed him away. When this happened three or four times with different men, she reached out to me for help.

Do you see yourself when reading this? Do you often regret that you had sexual encounters, and do you feel guilty that you got some pleasure? Well, you're not alone! Research[10] suggests that around 50 percent of women will regret their hookups and feel ashamed of their encounters because they feel ashamed for being sluts and being disrespected by men or society. In contrast, only 30 percent of men will regret their hookups—but not because of shame. Their reasons are different: because the woman didn't perform well, they didn't

---

[10] Elizabeth L. Paul and Kristen A. Hayes, "The Casualties of 'Casual' Sex: A Qualitative Exploration of the Phenomenology of College Students' Hookups," *Journal of Social and Personal Relationships* 19, no. 5 (October 2002): 639–61, https://doi.org/10.1177/0265407502195006.

find her very attractive, or they thought they could have done better. Quite a different perspective.

To be fair, women are absolutely right to be concerned about societal judgments. Although sexual attitudes have shifted over the last half century, research suggests that there are still many unfair societal judgments about women who enjoy hookups. A study[11] done by the University of Illinois in 2013 shows that there are big double standards about human sexuality and who should—or should not—be having casual sex. Over 20,000 students from twenty-two different universities across the United States were asked if they would lose respect for a man or a woman who "hooked up a lot," and guess what? Twenty-eight percent of men said "yes" for a woman but "no" for a man. As you might assume, double standards are usually employed in stricter, more male-dominated societies to exercise greater control over women's behavior.[12]

If you are one of those women who are brave enough to ask for pleasure and enjoy yourself, don't destroy this wonderful quality by being ashamed of who you are the day after. Sex feels good. It's fun, and we all need closeness.

---

[11] Rachel Allison and Barbara J. Risman, "A Double Standard for 'Hooking Up': How Far Have We Come toward Gender Equality?" *Social Science Research* 42, no. 5 (September 2013): 1191–1206, https://doi.org/10.1016/j.ssresearch.2013.04.006.

[12] Adina Nack, "Bad Girls and Fallen Women: Chronic STD Diagnoses as Gateways to Tribal Stigma," *Symbolic Interaction* 25, no. 4 (November 2002): 463–85, https://doi.org/10.1525/si.2002.25.4.463; Elizabeth A. Armstrong, Laura T. Hamilton, Elizabeth M. Armstrong, and J. Lotus Seeley, "'Good Girls.'" *Social Psychology Quarterly* 77, no. 2 (May 28, 2014): 100–122, https://doi.org/10.1177/0190272514521220.

I learned about double standards the hard way. After my explorative one-night stands as a teenager, often I'd never hear from my partners again. Later, I'd hear around town that these men were being praised by their friends. I wasn't hurt at the loss of their immature cocks. Instead, I felt more surprised and angrier at the judgment in society: days, weeks, and even months of approaching me with a goal of getting into my pants turned into ignoring me literally overnight. They were the heroes, and I was the slut.

Later, I left the small town I grew up in with hopes of finding a place where people were less judgmental so I could enjoy the gift of my creative sexuality without shame. Even today, I still advocate for a shame-free environment for both women and men. I will continue to strongly disagree with judgments against any kind of sexuality and the "slut vs. stud" attitude. Even though sexual attitudes have shifted over the last half century, research suggests that there are still many unfair societal judgments about women who enjoy hookups.

Tip #24:
ACCEPT WHAT YOU
CAN'T CHANGE

You don't have any control over another human being, and if he's not into you, you can't change it. The more you try, the worse it will get, so just accept it and move on.

Before I came to this conclusion, I spent a lot of valuable energy on many worthless and weird men just because I wanted to make things work. I was often pushy; I didn't take no for an answer, and many times I got angry and we ended up in a fight. Sometimes I wouldn't stop texting him because I was pissed off and he wasn't responsive. I didn't care if he thought I was a psycho—at that point I just wanted to annoy him. I would call from hidden numbers. I would text from the internet or Google Voice numbers. Once, I even placed an online dating ad with his picture and his real phone number. I simply couldn't let go of him telling me no.

Today I'm wiser and much calmer, but the transformation took some time. The first time I realized that it's beautiful to go with the flow and accept things as they are was at the Burning Man Festival in 2008. Through a tough week in the desert when not everything went well, I realized that sometimes it's good to accept discomfort and let things naturally unfold. Sometimes you have to believe that the Universe has your back and that there is a reason for everything.

A few years ago, in my early thirties, I did my first ayahuasca ceremony and understood what absolute acceptance and letting go meant. It was the first time I totally let go of all control and accepted that there was nothing I could do to change the situation. I knew I would be ridiculously high for the next six hours, accepting whatever the medicine led me through. I wasn't the same when I came back from the jungle. I loved myself more. I respected and appreciated my time more because I realized it's not infinite. I was picking the right battles based on a simple rule I'm still using today: "What you can't accept, change. What you can't change, accept."

When it comes to hookups, if he never texts, who cares? It wasn't meant to be. There could be thousands of reasons why, and you don't need to know all of them. It's probably better that way. If he texts you, keep the communication simple, and reply without overthinking. If he's the one, the conversation will flow organically.

So why am I mentioning all this here? Because I want you to save your wonderful energy for people and things that matter. Haven't you wanted to visit your parents for lunch so many Sundays, but you didn't have time to do it? Didn't you want to hit that new gym or a barre class, but you never had time? Do it. Perhaps you wanted to call your granddad, who would appreciate hearing your voice more than anything. Or maybe your job is sucking all the life out of you, so focus some energy on finding a better gig. Lastly, don't forget there is one person you need to care for the most. As Derek Walcott says in his poem[13] *Love after Love*, "You will love again the stranger who was yourself."

---

[13] Derek Walcott, "Love After Love," in *Collected Poems 1948–1984* (New York: Farrar, Straus, and Giroux, 1987).

Part 2

. . . .

THE PROS AND CONS
OF HOOKUPS

Casual sex: many men enjoy it, and women can, too, if they can handle it. What are the pros and cons of hookups, then? What should we keep in mind? To write this chapter, I spoke to some girlfriends and female clients of mine and asked them to share their takes and experiences on hookups. I also dug into the research about the advantages of hookups—but to my surprise, the resources were limited. This topic seems to be largely unexplored territory, making the real-life experiences shared here all the more valuable.

TO HOOK UP OR NOT TO HOOK UP?

Sexual hookups may leave more strings attached than many lovers might first assume. There are some people who love them and some who don't. The latest research[14] has shown that women who have a healthy view about sex, as well as those who are open to exploration, will experience more positive feelings around their own hookups. In contrast, the individuals who have more reserved behavior toward casual sex will experience more regret, shame, and other negative emotions after playing with someone.

Let's discuss some pros and cons of one-night stands and casual hookups so you're aware of the potential risks of these encounters. I want you to be aware of what you are getting yourself into, so you can answer an age-old question: Is it better to date and wait? Or to go ahead and get laid?

Pro #1:
GENERAL POSITIVE FEELINGS

Flirting, seducing, and playing are…well, fun. Humans love sex because thinking about it or having it helps our brains to release dopamine. Dopamine is a feel-good neurotransmitter involved in

---

[14] Zhana Vrangalova and Anthony D. Ong, "Who Benefits From Casual Sex? The Moderating Role of Sociosexuality," *Social Psychological and Personality Science* 5, no. 8 (June 6, 2014): 883–91, https://doi.org/10.1177/1948550614537308.

mood, motivation, and attention, and it boosts learning and movement. It's a chemical that not only helps us see the possible rewards but also motivates us to take action toward them. For the time being, casual sex gives us temporary happiness. In fact,[15] first-year college women experienced positive feelings following hookups that were associated with social connection, the ability to explore their sexuality and be intimate with someone, and simple fun/enjoyment. Also, when we're sexually stimulated, it's easy to forget the world around us. It's often difficult to switch off from our daily routine or to forget the stress associated with work and responsibilities. Then, suddenly there's this new person we're meeting with whom we can have light and refreshing conversations! We quickly find that we're happy, laughing, flirting, and enjoying the moment. (For the positivity to linger, keep it light. Don't over-analyze the hookup the next day so you can keep your good mood going.)

Pro #2:
NOVELTY IS EXCITING

S ex is fun, and it should offer some form of pleasure. Although having sex with someone you don't know doesn't guarantee a massive orgasm, we are usually so excited because of the unknown and the novelty that there's the potential to have a great time even

---

[15] Robyn L. Shepardson, Jennifer L. Walsh, Kate B. Carey, and Michael P. Carey, "Benefits of Hooking Up: Self-Reports from First-Year College Women," *International Journal of Sexual Health* 28, no. 3 (July 2, 2016): 216–20, https://doi.org/10.1080/19317611.2016.1178677.

without coming. Frankly, how many times have you reached orgasm with a first-timer? How many times did you have sex without orgasm, but you still enjoyed it? Many women are used to that. It's not only because of the fact[16] that 75 percent of women can't reach penetrative orgasm, but it's also because most men will not lick you on the first play date. Many forums and casual surveys[17] found that women consider sex good when they don't have pain! Men consider it to be good sex when they have an orgasm.

It's not fair, I know. But we also know that after some time spent flirting with the object of our desire and fantasizing, we can have a great time hooking up! And novelty is always exciting. In one study[18] of 118 female college students, 58 percent stated that their desire to hook up was associated with the thrill of spontaneity. Additionally, researchers[19] found that there is a decrease in both arousal and desire as your partner becomes more familiar with you. Conversely, there's an increase in desire and arousal, for both men and women, when your partner is someone new. We need new experiences that keep us

---

[16] Michael Castleman, "The Most Important Sexual Statistic," *Psychology Today*, last modified March 16, 2009, https://www.psychologytoday.com/us/blog/all-about-sex/200903/the-most -important-sexual-statistic.

[17] Lili Loofbourow, "The Female Price of Male Pleasure," *The Week*, last modified January 25, 2018, https://theweek.com/articles/749978/female-price-male-pleasure.

[18] Justin R. Garcia, Chris Reiber, Sean G. Massey, and Ann M. Merriwether, "Sexual Hookup Culture: A Review," *Review of General Psychology* 16, no. 2 (June 2012): 161–76, https://doi.org/10.1037 /a0027911.

[19] Heather Morton and Boris B. Gorzalka, "Role of Partner Novelty in Sexual Functioning: A Review," *Journal of Sex & Marital Therapy* 41, no. 6 (October 28, 2014): 593–609, https://doi .org/10.1080/0092623x.2014.958788.

alive! And what can be better than to feel alive?

Pro #3:
SELF-ESTEEM BOOST

As humans, it makes us feel good to be chased and desired. The attention, compliments, and sometimes begging for more boost our egos. Many women complain that they get annoyed when a particular man is texting them or asking them out, but deep inside, it's flattering! When we have a crush on someone and agree on a date, the preparation is fun and makes us feel good. The fantasizing about what we will wear, how we will look, and how he will undress us makes us feel good. Enjoy the attention that you're giving yourself and getting from your seducer.

But what if you just met him in a bar and decided to fuck him immediately that evening? No problem! Getting someone into your bed to devour your body is a great boost to your self-esteem, not only for men but also for women. You don't have to take my word for it alone. There's even research[20] that supports it.

---

[20] Vrangalova found that among 371 college students who identified themselves as sexually permissive, those who engaged in casual sex on a regular basis, reported higher levels of self-esteem as well as lower rates of anxiety and depression. This was in comparison to those who rated themselves as more permissive but failed to engage in casual sex. In other words, it gave their self-esteem a boost to know they could achieve what they set out to do—have sex!

Zhana Vrangalova, "Hooking Up and Psychological Well-Being in College Students: Short-Term Prospective Links Across Different Hookup Definitions," *The Journal of Sex Research* 52, no. 5 (July 29, 2014): 485–98, https://doi.org/10.1080/00224499.2014.910745.

Pro #4:

NO EXPECTATIONS

I know that men might seem to be the ones who don't want commitment. But times, they are a-changin', and there are more and more women who actually don't want to be in a long-term relationship, get married, and/or have children right away. Committed relationships are beautiful but bring more responsibilities, and they are not for everyone. In today's culture, many women also want to focus on their careers and be independent. In fact, the median age for a first marriage has risen from twenty for women in 1960 to twenty-seven now. For men, it's gone from twenty-three in 1960 to twenty-nine today.[21]

What's more, fully half of single adults in a Pew Research Center survey[22] from August 2020 indicated that they are not looking for a relationship or to date. And of those who are dating, half of them were open to having either a committed relationship or just casually dating. As for gender differences, it was single men who were more likely to be looking for a steady relationship of some kind. Only 38 percent of women said they were looking for commitment versus 61

---

[21] Wendy Wang and Kim Parker, "Record Share of Americans Have Never Married," *Pew Research Center*, last modified September 24, 2014, https://www.pewsocialtrends.org/2014/09/24/record-share-of-americans-have-never-married/.

[22] Anna Brown, "Nearly Half of U.S. Adults Say Dating Has Gotten Harder for Most People in the Last 10 Years," *Pew Research Center*, last modified August 20, 2020, https://www.pewsocial trends.org/2020/08/20/nearly-half-of-u-s-adults-say-dating-has-gotten-harder-for-most-people -in-the-last-10-years/.

percent of men. This gap was particularly apparent in older singles.

Surprised? Me too, as this finding is exactly the opposite of what we all believe: the cliché that men just want to fuck around and have no commitment. The most common reason for women not wanting to be in a serious relationship was mainly that they had more important priorities in their lives. My guess is that the results could also be influenced by the COVID-19 pandemic that struck our world in 2020. I remember that many good male friends were texting me while stuck in quarantine, going crazy from boredom and no sex. Men seem to struggle more without a sexual partner, especially when they are used to having casual sex often. The funniest part was that even players who claimed they would never marry were promising to find steady partners ASAP.

Another reason for not being in a relationship was feeling less pressure from society and the families of the participants to get married and have a family. Thanks to that, you won't feel obligated to marry the first guy you sleep with and won't be ashamed to be thirty-plus and single. This allows you to explore sexually more often and then to move on. My tip on moving on more easily is to make it clear to yourself that the sex you're about to have is just for fun. Remind yourself that even though nature makes you feel otherwise, you will avoid getting fooled by the feeling that you're in love and want to form a bond.

My next tip is to communicate your desire for an NSA relationship with your beau, making sure that you're on the same page. This will also weed out controlling and jealous men who will want to own you right after you sleep with them. Been there, done that. A couple of casual sex experiences turned into an unnecessary drama after the gentleman realized he was not the only one I was playing with. I got some nasty phone calls and visits as a result. That's not to mention the slut-shaming coming from his hurt ego.

A shocking fact I discovered about slut-shaming is that the men who are most likely to disrespect women who like hookups are the men with the same interest! So basically, the sluttier the man is, the more he is going to slut-shame you—the ultimate double standard. This isn't just an act of total hypocrisy—it is also totally detrimental to their sexual interests.

All told, life is too short. Be clear and strict about your independence. Most men will love your honesty and directness. Plus, who wouldn't want to get laid without drama?

Pro #5:
A BREAK FROM YOUR VIBRATOR

Masturbation is fun, but sometimes you just want to take a break from your vibrator and feel the real meat instead. It's good to practice different movements, thrusts, and pleasuring techniques on your own, so you can then communicate them to your partner, sure. But the fact is that sex toys won't give you the feeling of connection that having a real human next to you does. Take a break from your vibrator and put the knowledge you have gained about yourself and your genitals into practice.

Pro #6:
AFTER-SEX GLOW

Sex releases endorphins, chemicals that boost estrogen levels, which enhances skin elasticity and collagen production. Did it ever happen to you that you came to work or met friends after a night full of sex and everyone said that you're glowing? It's true! Orgasms make you look hot! Your face is glowing, your skin is radiant, and your breasts are—well, yeah, perkier. Some women experience fuller hair, almost like a dry shampoo effect. And no, I'm not talking about JBF hair here. When I was happily fucked, people used to tell me how great my hair looked. You can be floating on post-orgasm bliss for around forty-eight hours. Scientists[23] have actually documented this effect. They believe it occurs to facilitate bonding, but you can use it to your advantage. You will look sexier and healthier, and you can take advantage of this attraction and line up your next lover, if you choose.

The bottom line? Even if nothing else works out after the hookup, you got a beauty boost similar to a day in the spa.

---

[23] Andrea L. Meltzer, Anastasia Makhanova, Lindsey L. Hicks, Juliana E. French, James K. McNulty, and Thomas N. Bradbury, "Quantifying the Sexual Afterglow: The Lingering Benefits of Sex and Their Implications for Pair-Bonded Relationships," *Psychological Science* 28, no. 5 (March 16, 2017): 587–98, https://doi.org/10.1177/0956797617691361.

Pro #7:
TRY OUT YOUR SECRET KINKS

Some of us have sexual kinks that are considered outside the norm. To that end, I have a different opinion on the norm: I consider everything normal. Unfortunately, there's still our society and its rules that put the "different" ones into a "weird" category. Many people are ashamed of their outside-of-the-box fetishes and fantasies, and they couldn't imagine doing them with someone they are seriously dating or married to. You might ask yourself why, but the answer to that is rather complex. (I cover this in-depth in my book *Play with Power*.)

When I worked as a dominatrix, I had many men who would dream about being restrained, humiliated, or pegged (to have a woman perform anal sex on them with a strap-on), but they would never have the courage to ask for these acts from their own partners. The reason is fear and shame. Interestingly, they had no issues with sharing this secret with a dominatrix, escort, or casual hookup. They didn't care so much about what those ladies thought, as they were strangers to them.

You can tell your casual hookup about your dirty little secrets and ask him to play out your fantasy. Do you like, or have fantasies about, sleeping with men, women, or transgender people? Do you want to be gang-banged, restrained, and deep-throated like a little slut? Go for it. It's far easier to share these fantasies with your hookup than with your steady Eddie.

Here's a pro tip: tell your casual sex partner what you desire and have all your toys ready. He might be too shy to do it, but if this person is the same kind of freak as you, you will have a perfect night!

Pro #8:
SEX GIVES YOU POWER

Being sexually independent is empowering. The babe who isn't ashamed of her own sexuality doesn't have a problem asking men for pleasure, and she will enjoy sex fully like a true goddess. Throughout history and even today, men are scared of female sexuality because the biggest male weakness is the irresistible desire for sex. To keep women under their control, they came up with their unfair ideas about how women must be faithful, reserved, and monogamous —which actually protects them from losing their minds and the fight. (I will get back to this topic in much greater detail in Part 3 of this book.)

Times are changing, and women are regaining control of their sexuality. Even still, there's a long way to go to achieve perfect equality. Having the right to have sex anytime you want and being able to freely ask for it gives you *power*. The self-esteem boost you get through sex gives you *power*. Have fun, ladies—the power is within you!

Pro #9:

YOU HAVE FREEDOM

The real beauty of casual sex is that you officially can't hurt anyone's feelings. The caveat here is that unofficially, you can…but nobody can directly blame you as long as you communicate your wants and needs (don't forget!). Literally, after the act, you can take your stuff and go home (or tell him to leave because you need to sleep).

I personally couldn't stay overnight with a casual hookup. I would set myself up for disaster and a completely sleepless night. I have no problem having sex with a man whose name I barely know, but sleeping with him in one bed and waking up next to him? No way—that's something special I reserve only for a romantic partner whom I trust and feel comfortable with. I don't want to risk falling asleep and waking up with my legs and arms restrained or a finger in my anus. (Yeah, it almost happened. But thankfully, I woke up and boxed that asshole down to the ground!)

Besides being used and abused while you sleep, the man next to you is a stranger. You don't know his sleeping habits. What if he snores? What if he has nightmares and moves around, screams, or calls for his mom in the middle of the night? He could even sleepwalk! No way—too many unknowns. I will take all my stuff, kiss him goodbye, and leave for the safety of my home.

You may be wondering: *But Lia, what if the date doesn't go well and I feel like leaving?* You sure can! Take advantage of the freedom that hooking up provides you. Remember, once you're in a committed relationship, things just get more complicated.

Pro #10:
IT'S A LEARNING EXPERIENCE

I'm sure you've heard the saying, "We met for a reason—either you're a blessing or a lesson." Hookups, no matter how they end up, are always a learning experience. You can learn anything from new sexual positions to techniques and practices, but it also goes much deeper than that. You will learn how to attract and seduce a man. You can observe how the man seduced you and see what you enjoyed about his techniques. What did you like? What didn't you like? Was it his sense of humor? The way he looked at you? His voice?

You will also learn about yourself and your attachment style.[24] During early childhood, we're forming different behaviors and reactions through the relationships with our primary caregivers. These behaviors and habits are later projected on our romantic relationships. How did the experience move you? How did you manage to get out of uncomfortable situations? Were you able to let go? Or perhaps,

---

[24] R. Chris Fraley, "Adult Attachment Theory and Research: A Brief Overview," accessed May 12, 2021 http://labs.psychology.illinois.edu/~rcfraley/attachment.htm.

was your needy ego upset for a longer time than necessary? What would you like to get better at? Not giving a fuck? Letting go? Being kinder? Remember, growth only comes from pain. If you want to learn and grow on a personal and spiritual level, hookups can help you do just that!

Con #1:
PREGNANCY AND STIS

Bringing home a souvenir from a one-night stand is a real risk that you must avoid. Sure, you can get pregnant with your regular partner, but this situation gets more dramatic when you don't know the person well. They might be nice and clean, but they might not. If they sleep with you without a condom, they're probably doing it with other people too. Remember, people are creatures of habit, and if they feel it's safe to sleep with you bare, how many others were there in the past? In fact,[25] 3 percent of hookups result in an STI, and research has shown that hookup behavior is a significant predictor for STIs.

What if you get pregnant? With a beau whom you literally know nothing about, it can be a real disaster. Abortion can be emotionally and physically exhausting, so no fun should lead to that. If you get

---

[25] Robyn L. Fielder, Jennifer L. Walsh, Kate B. Carey, and Michael P. Carey, "Sexual Hookups and Adverse Health Outcomes: A Longitudinal Study of First-Year College Women," *The Journal of Sex Research* 51, no. 2 (December 18, 2013): 131–44, https://doi.org/10.1080/00224499.2013.848255.

pregnant with your regular partner, it's easier to work together to decide what to do. But with a casual hookup, there are just too many unknowns. So please, be safe and responsible, and let the passion carry you away *after* you put the condom on.

Con #2:
SOCIAL STIGMA AND REGRETS

There's never a perfect scenario for a woman. Your dress is too short, or your outfit is too boxy and masculine. Your hair is too long or too short. Your nail polish is too red. You're not a good mother because you're working too much, or you're a lazy housewife who lets your husband do all the work!

As a woman, you're stigmatized for everything. Unfortunately, the harshest stigmas of all are reserved for your sexual behaviors. The culture we live in has a norm of sexual monogamy, and sadly, still holds on to the idea of women being good girls. This has historically meant either waiting until marriage or sleeping around with fewer partners than men.

Cultural influence as a whole is powerful, helps us survive as a species, and provides a superstructure for how we behave in different circumstances. As we grow and learn, we come to understand the expected behaviors for any given role. We strive to behave appropriately often without realizing it. Why? Think about it: in many cultures even today, ostracization can mean death. That's a powerful influence over individual behavior, and it's why stigmas of any kind work to help keep people in line.

Even today, one of the biggest fears people have is not being accepted and/or being left out from their respective social group(s). Many people commit suicide just because of the cultural pressure and anxiety of being excluded. This mindfuck is very powerful!

Have you ever liked a man, and were really horny, but you chose not to have sex with him because of the fear of judgment and of being excluded? Or have you opted to have fun and not give a fuck about what other people say, only to end up lonely and full of regrets when people pointed fingers at you?

I'm not surprised if that happened because judgments are commonplace in a stuck-up society. Not only that, but there's research supporting your feelings! In a recent survey[26] that asked participants how they felt after their most recent hookup, "women said they felt more lonely, unhappy, rejected, regretful, felt more negative feelings about themselves and were more concerned about being negatively judged by others."

This means that ladies, if you're not a master of "no fucks given,"

---

[26] Ryan Anderson, "Gender Differences in Casual Sex," *Psychology Today*, last modified April 2, 2020, https://www.psychologytoday.com/us/blog/the-mating-game/202004/gender -differences-in-casual-sex.

there's a chance you'll spend weeks regretting your last casual sex experience, together with other negative feelings.

Con #3:
AWKWARDNESS

This is really an…awkward one. Have you gotten hit with a wave of sudden passion and slept with someone, only later to realize you shouldn't have done it? Maybe it was your classmate, teacher, coworker, boss, long-term friend…you name it. I even heard a story from a girlfriend who slipped and slept with her next-door neighbor. She shared how weird it became for her to bring other men to her house, hoping she wouldn't run into him. Yikes.

When casual sex happens in an inappropriate manner and you are expected to see your lover on a regular basis, things can get really awkward. I've heard stories of women having sex with their boss at a Christmas party, classmates while doing their homework, a student and a teacher in the biology cabinet—and, of course, colleagues on a work trip.

After these kinds of encounters, you're obviously dealing with much greater repercussions than when you sleep with a stranger from Tinder. You can get fired, ruin friendships, or have all kinds of other daily drama.

Con #4:

TOO REPETITIVE

Although novelty is usually exciting, you can get bored with that, too. Even if you sleep with a different man, there's usually a similar story. You meet up for dinner, drinks, and go to his place or yours. Sometimes it could be a hotel. Later that night or in the morning, you part ways feeling disappointed because it's the same as it was with the other guys: usually there's alcohol involved, you have a massive hangover, and your head is swirling with contradictory thoughts. Yeah, it was good, but…

It's difficult to have romantic and loving hookups. Things must stay in the department of casual interactions and no-strings-attached sex, and *both* parties want to keep those boundaries clear. Putting in an extra effort with lovemaking could come off as clingy, and casual lovers try to avoid such sensibilities. I know it's not easy to make love to a stranger, but I've heard from experienced players that sex without love and genuine emotion is empty and gets boring after a while.

Con #5:

BAD REPUTATION IF YOU
OVERLAP CIRCLES

If you've made it to this point, you obviously know I have nothing against a woman who's sleeping around. I'm glad she's brave enough to explore and have fun! But if this is you, pay attention: if you overlap circles and lovers find out about each other, it can limit your dating prospects and increase the slut-shaming that is fueled by the aforementioned double standards around casual sex. This bad-mouthing can ruin your potential to find a serious relationship …although you surely won't have a lack of lovers.

A tip for the ladies: if you want to sleep around, make sure you're picking your lovers from different circles or choosing men who are discreet. Tell them to shut up. If they don't, it will be the last time they can taste your pussy. You can easily find out through social media if your two lovers know each other. As unjust as it is, being discreet can prevent you from building a bad reputation that can be difficult to overcome. There are also men who are sex-positive and don't care, but make sure that's who you really want to date.

Con #6:
BROKEN HEARTS

There are only two forces that we can't fight: Mother Nature and love. Even after one or two nights of passionate sex, there's a chance that one of you will fall in love and then get hurt. Your lover might fall in love with you, and you'll be in an uncomfortable situation when you have to tell him that you don't want to see him again. Or you might be the one feeling the butterflies in your stomach and heat all over your body when you're thinking of him. This book might help you to understand what's happening to you when you sexually bond with someone and how you can do your best to fight nature with a rational mind (it's difficult, as you know).

My tip here is to be intuitive and know the best time to stop the affair. Do you feel he's in love with you, and you can't reciprocate? Or do you feel that you're falling in love with him, and he's not there yet? Stop it as soon as you can. The longer you linger in the feelings of love and fantasy, the harder it will be to let go.

Con #7:
NO ORGASM

If you're hoping to have a fantastic sexual experience while hooking up, you might want to revise those expectations. In a large study[27] of over 12,000 undergraduates from seventeen different colleges, researchers found that only 10 percent of the women who engaged in hookups achieved orgasm. That compares with 31 percent of men who achieved orgasm. For this study, researchers identified a hookup as a wide range of sexual activities, such as kissing, oral sex, and penetrative intercourse.

---

[27] Justin R. Garcia, Chris Reiber, Sean G. Massey, and Ann M. Merriwether, "Sexual Hookup Culture: A Review," *Review of General Psychology* 16, no. 2 (June 2012): 161–76, https://doi.org/10.1037/a0027911.

It's always harder to reach an orgasm when you don't know your partner well or their sexual preferences. What turns them on? How do they like to be touched? What movements, positions, and special caresses can help them get there? While you might be turned on by the novelty of sex with a stranger, the reality is often less sexy than the fantasy.

Con #8:
SHAME

Do you remember that moment when you came home after a hot date, still smelling like sex, and instead of feeling totally satisfied and happy, you began questioning what you had done? "I acted like a slut again!" you might say into the mirror, while looking at your messed-up hair. Shame is common in these cases and is detrimental to our well-being. Of course, preferably, we do things we won't feel ashamed of later on—but when it comes to sex and females, it gets tricky. Shame is so deeply rooted in our psyches that there should be no surprise that this dark little voice of your teacher, parent, priest, or schoolmate still chatters on deep inside your head. "Bad girl! You are naughty, and you shouldn't be," it says. My advice? Tell this voice to shut up!

Con #9:

SEXUAL VICTIMIZATION

You never know whom you're meeting up with when you hook up on Tinder or meet someone online, and that's also true when you meet someone for casual sex in any other setting. Unsurprisingly, there is an association between hooking up and sexual victimization (i.e., unwanted sexual behavior). In one study,[28] a full 25 percent of college students who had hookup experience reported unwanted sex during their college years.

This is due in part to the nature of a hookup and how it can lead men to misperceive a woman's feelings about sex. Men and women differ in their expectations for how far a hookup should go, and each sex commonly overestimates the other gender's comfort level regarding the appropriateness of sexual behaviors during a hookup. Added to this is the fact that you don't know him very well and you're probably not going to be as comfortable discussing your sexual preferences during the hookup. Add alcohol to the mix, and you've got the makings of an unwanted sexual encounter.

My advice: on sexually driven dates and in such environments, always be very, *very* clear about your expectations and any behavior you

---

[28] Robyn L. Fielder, Jennifer L. Walsh, Kate B. Carey, and Michael P. Carey, "Sexual Hookups and Adverse Health Outcomes: A Longitudinal Study of First-Year College Women," *The Journal of Sex Research* 51, no. 2 (December 18, 2013): 131–44, https://doi.org/10.1080/00224499 .2013.848255.

consider to be out of line. Shame has no place in the conversation about establishing boundaries. It is your body and your soul, and you know how bad an unwanted sexual experience can be for your mental health and well-being.

Men get mixed signals when women are flirty. For them it might mean an evening of wild sex, but for you it means cuddling up and having your back rubbed or pussy licked. Tell him your boundaries straightforwardly when things are heating up, and don't wait until he's all hot and horny. It could be more difficult then. You can say: "I'm into you and I would like to be intimate with you tonight, but I do not feel like having penetration/sleeping with you/getting naked quite yet. How about a nice back massage/hand job/oral sex/kissing?" (Fill in whatever your boundary is.) You can also add: "I hope you can respect my boundaries so we can both have fun."

If he is too pushy, you can always say, "This pressure doesn't seem right for me, and I might have to leave." But if he isn't respecting your boundary in the first place, it is time to go home no matter what. If you don't want to go into the details and ruin the moment, just tell him that you would like to play using a safe word, let's say "blueberry," and that you will use it to put a stop to anything you don't like if it starts to happen. Here's how this would look in practice: if he's trying to take your pants off and you're not into it, simply kiss him and say, "Blueberry. Another time, babe, I'm not there yet."

Good luck and stay safe.

Con #10:
STALKER DANGER

A recent study[29] examined sexual harassment and stalking among adolescents. The researchers found that both adolescents who engage in sexual harassment or stalking and those who have experienced problems with a stalker are more likely to have had casual sex. In other words, the study found that a person's preferences for casual sex could increase their risk of being harassed by a stalker. It's possible that this is related to the fact[30] that someone who engages in casual sex receives more sexual solicitations in general, as opposed to someone who does not have casual sex. This can also be a factor in the risk of sexual victimization.

That's not to say that the victim is at fault. There's nothing wrong with a preference for casual sex, and if you like to hook up, you should be able to do that on your own terms without fear of stalking or sexual victimization. But it's important to understand the risks involved so that you can keep yourself safe.

---

[29] Leif Edward Ottesen Kennair and Mons Bendixen, "Sociosexuality as Predictor of Sexual Harassment and Coercion in Female and Male High School Students," *Evolution and Human Behavior* 33, no. 5 (September 2012): 479–90. https://doi.org/10.1016/j.evolhumbehav.2012.01.001.

[30] Ottesen Kennair and Bendixen, "Sociosexuality as Predictor of Sexual Harassment and Coercion in Female and Male High School Students," 479–90.

TIPS FOR STAYING SAFE
WHILE HOOKING UP

To help prevent either stalking or sexual victimization, be sure to document your hookup's Tinder information or get a name or photo of him. Additionally, it can help to ask questions before agreeing to meet. You should definitely Google his name and image to see if he's part of other websites, businesses, etc. A video call before you go on a real date with someone you've met online is a good way to do this.

When you do meet, start out in a public place, and stay there until you feel comfortable going someplace more private. Let a friend know that you're with someone and where you are going for the hookup. If you meet him in a public place and decide to go elsewhere, let someone know. Be sure to have your cell phone with you, and make sure it is fully charged.

Stay in control of your transportation. Don't go in his car. You drive your car, let him drive his, or take a cab or public transportation. Do not let him pick you up by your house. Then he will know where you live, and that can get really risky if things don't go well. If he assures you it's OK to drive with him, be honest and follow your gut. If you sense any red flags coming from your date, don't be afraid to simply end it and leave.

I will never forget a potentially dangerous date I went on in New York. I met a man online, and we had some interesting exchanges. He was older, single, and lived in a beautiful house about an hour north of Boston. He drove to New York to meet up with me one evening. I don't know if I was out of my mind giving him my address, but I told him to pick me up. He was there about half an hour before our date and sat in the car, observing my house. When I came down, we drove to the restaurant, and I immediately felt like his energy was weird. There was some kind of pain and anger that he was trying to hide in his fake smile. I felt uncomfortable, and when I heard he drove from Boston just to see me for dinner, I felt bad to tell him goodbye and leave.

Dinner was painful. He complained the whole time about his life, health, and the pain he was going through. He was much older than in his pictures (I think mid-sixties). At the end of dinner, he requested I pack a bag and go to his house with him for the weekend. I politely refused. He insisted on driving me home and kept trying to persuade me to come with him: "It will be a lovely weekend. I'm so lonely there. I can show you around, and we can go kayaking or surfing." I kept explaining that I couldn't go, and maybe next time.

At some point he grabbed my breast and started yelling at me about why the heck he drove to New York for nothing. I pushed his hand aside and politely said that we could plan something for another time. His face became deeply creased and aggressive. His eyes were glassy, and I was awaiting foam at his mouth or him biting me or taking a knife out of his pocket. Thankfully, we were almost back to my apartment, and in front of my building he escalated for the last time as I was leaving the car, screaming, "Whore, you wasted my time!"

Then he left. Thank God a doorman was already opening the door for me and asking if everything was all right. I can tell you I had some worrisome weeks after this, and I have never met a man in front of my house again or let one drive me.

If you want to feel more secure about the man you're meeting, ask him for his real name before your date and try to do a background check on him. You can sign up for a background check website and find out if he has any criminal history, where he lives, and if he's had traffic violations or even debts. There are some complex websites that will provide you with detailed information for a membership fee.

Set Strict Boundaries

Be aware of the effects that alcohol or drugs have on you and avoid becoming so intoxicated that your judgment or alertness is impaired. Never leave your drink or your personal items unattended. Remember, no matter how charming he is, you don't know him, and while sexual assault is rare with hookups, you need to take all precautions to stay safe. Only accept drinks from the bartender or wait staff and keep your personal items with you at all times. If anything feels "off" to you, just end the date and leave. Don't feel like you can't do that.

Lastly, as I mentioned in the discussion of sexual victimization, talk candidly with your date about your expectations and comfort level for various sexual behaviors. When discussing your boundaries, use words and a tone of voice that are clear and not sexually suggestive.

There's a "no" that might sound like you're hedging and a "no" that leaves no doubt. Women often say a "no" that sounds more like "yes" because they use a flirty and playful tone. Men get confused and, when it's said quietly, might not even hear you. Be clear and strict when you say NO, so he immediately understands. Preferably, discuss your boundaries before you get into an uncomfortable situation when he is horny and upset that you backed off.

Know your STI status and ask him his. Regardless of what he says, insist on a condom. Don't feel ashamed to ask these kinds of questions. It's also important to know that, while the laws vary in different states and countries, knowingly engaging in sex with someone when you are aware that you have an STI and not informing them about it can result in criminal charges if they contract the disease from you. In some states in the US, it's still possible to be criminally charged if your partner becomes infected, even if you *do* inform them and they agree to have sex with you anyway. Make sure you know your rights and the laws where you're located, and communicate with any potential hookups about this important topic. And, just to reiterate—always use protection when hooking up. It's just not worth the risk.

It is not your fault

No matter what, you don't deserve to be attacked while seeking an intimate connection. It doesn't matter whether you let your guard down or did everything possible to stay safe—if you are assaulted, IT IS NOT YOUR FAULT. You are never to blame if you are sexually assaulted. If it happens, report it to the police and tell them if you were using a dating app to meet up with the perpetrator. The police should notify the dating app so they can assist with the investigation and help keep him from hurting someone else.

Don't shower until investigators have had a chance to collect evidence from you. Call someone you love and trust to help you through the investigation and support you emotionally. If you're scared to talk to a friend or family member for fear of being blamed or shamed, please find a psychotherapist you can talk to.

Part 3

· ·

THE HISTORY AND SCIENCE AROUND HOOKUPS

Since when are we hooking up? Some might think hooking up is a trend of the nineties or the early twenty-first century. I thought that, too. Once I dug more into the history, though, I realized I was wrong. Hooking up was normal sexual behavior for our ancestors living in hunter-and-gatherer societies. These guys had a pretty open-minded, polyamorous view of life, and sex was available to anyone. Women weren't slut-shamed for enjoying their bodies or pleasure with multiple men. Having sex with many at a time, or with someone else every day, was the norm. People weren't too greedy and didn't hoard food or belongings because, as they were always moving to places more abundant in food and resources, storage was not an option. (Remember that the wheel was not invented until 3500 B.C.)

It was a pretty equal time back then. Nobody had more than another, and whatever was caught was shared in the community so nobody starved. Sharing was caring, in the realms of both food and sex. Women weren't worried about being left alone without resources. When there was a lack of resources, everyone was affected. When a baby was born, the whole village or community took care of the baby. Since the child's father could have been pretty much anyone in the community, the children were used to growing up having multiple fathers.

But everything changed drastically with the arrival of agriculture, around 10,000 years ago. Men with more physical strength fought to own land and cattle. Stronger men had more resources, and the men without resources needed to work for the men with them to survive. Women, having less physical strength, were naturally disadvantaged and had to seek a man in order to have enough resources that she could survive. Soon after, women became the property of men and were expected to be sexually monogamous.

Why did men suddenly care about that? Certainly, jealousy and greed could have been one aspect of this change. What, though, made each man suddenly want to make sure he was taking care of his own offspring? The book *Sex at Dawn* makes an interesting argument to answer this question: men were putting so much labor into individual sections of land, rather than killing wild animals or gathering plants from a general area, that this gave them a sense of ownership and emotional investment in that land. As a result, they wanted to be sure that *their* children were the ones who would inherit the land, and that they weren't giving the land they'd worked so hard on away to other men's children.

Since women were susceptible to becoming pregnant, men forced women to be faithful. To achieve female monogamy, men used strategies like force and manipulation.

This possessive behavior began changing through the sexual revolution that happened in the Western world, especially in the United States, from the 1960s to the 1980s. The development of a contraceptive pill for women changed the attitudes toward hookups and casual sex. Women were able to have fun and enjoy sex without the dangers of unwanted pregnancy. Casual sex became more socially acceptable, but sadly, research shows that it remains much more acceptable for men than for women. Although we live in the twenty-first century and women are more emancipated than ever, no longer depend on men for survival, and can decide how we'd like to live our lives, we have a lot of work to do if we want to change the serious double standards around sex.

MEN VS. WOMEN
IN THE REALM OF HOOKUPS

L et me begin with a true story to which I was a witness. I know all the participants personally.

I wonder if Eduard will be there, Amelia asked herself on the way to the company's Christmas party. It was a cold December night, and she was dressed in a short skirt and over-the-knee leather boots—clothing she would normally never wear to the office, but which looked extra sexy for the occasion. It was her fifth year in Chicago. Running an HR team for an advertising company and her private psychotherapy office, she had barely any time to have a relationship. The cold air of the coming winter and thoughts about her single relationship status, which still remained over four years after her divorce, filled her with melancholy. There were many men who wanted this tall, skinny, blonde femme fatale of Scandinavian descent, but none of them could keep her engaged for too long.

That is, until about two months earlier, when she received a LinkedIn and phone number request from Eduard, a colleague she had met at a company dinner that night. He was hot, smart, and interesting. Their conversation lasted for over three hours, and she had a hard time not grabbing him and taking him home to have wild sex. But her boundaries kicked in, and she remembered she couldn't be intimate with her colleagues. Once he started texting, she became intrigued. There were moments when she wanted to tell him to fuck off because he wouldn't reply for days, and then his replies were lame, but suddenly he asked her an interesting question or sent her an erotic poem that made her head spin. This was nothing like what she was used to from other men.

She was glad he worked in a different department and they only ran into each other on rare occasions, but when they did, the air was electrifying. He showered her with smiles, offering her coffee, winking. *He's so into me*, thought Amelia, reconsidering her boundaries. The sexiest thing was his self-confidence that bordered on arrogance. Perhaps he was of Brazilian descent? Or Portuguese? She wanted to know more about him; she wanted to get more from him. Passion and fantasies were filling her head to the point that she was unable to focus on anything else in her life.

When she arrived at the Christmas party, it was in full effect. She walked across the big event room but couldn't see him. A bit relieved and disappointed at the same time, she sat in a chair and slowly sipped her wine. And then *she* walked in: a five-foot-tall, dark-skinned girl with a huge smile and beautiful white teeth, wearing a short skirt and over-the-knee boots. It was Bailey, a fun Puerto Rican student who had just joined the company as a content creator. They were definitely the most sexily dressed girls in the room, and Amelia decided to meet her in person.

Amelia stood up and walked straight to Bailey, who was smiling and drinking wine, already surrounded by three men. She wasn't the prettiest girl, but her happy, bubbly energy was intoxicating. After the introduction, Bailey freaked out knowing that Amelia's second gig was working on sexual and marital issues with couples. Still naïve on the subject of men, she was hunting and flirting all over the place, perhaps looking for the right one. She was the exact opposite of Amelia, who was an absolutely calm and introverted seductress. About ten years older, Amelia was filled with sexual confidence and didn't have a problem asking men for pleasure. She knew what she wanted and had her love life in control—or at least she thought so.

"I'm so glad I met a sex therapist! I will definitely need your help!" laughed Bailey, then continued flirting with the boys.

Months passed, and Amelia's desire for Mr. Secret was growing. She couldn't figure out the mixed signals he was sending her, keeping her emotional and confused. The many compliments and flattering messages that made her heart race had been exchanged for a diplomatic, almost cold demeanor while they were having lunch or coffee.

She was dying from desire—until the night when she succumbed to the passion and ended up in his bed. Passionate nights were followed by days of no replies. She could not wait to see him again, but he was cold and distant. Then, once together again, he gave her the deepest lovemaking and connection she could ever wish for. *This must be the one. We're such a great match!* she thought after every sex-filled night.

One Thursday, in the early evening, they met in a cozy restaurant to wine and dine. Amelia arrived first, excited for yet another hours-long arousing conversation, followed by the deepest lovemaking she had ever experienced. When he walked in, she knew he was coming, because every single head turned his direction. *What power he has!* she thought, and immediately got wet.

After many hours of sex, they usually fell asleep holding each other. But that night, he said he needed to leave earlier and go to one more meeting. He added that he needed to wake up at 5 a. m. to fly out of town. She felt disappointed, as it was supposed to be their special night. She felt anger, jealousy, and neediness, wanting more of this special man. She had skipped an important company networking event in order to see him, but she didn't blame him or beg him to stay.

"I will see you soon again," he said, giving her a long look that she wished would last for eternity. "You are lovely," he added and grabbed her around her thin waist, slowly and passionately kissing her. She melted into his eyes, and her skin was covered in goosebumps. She felt warmth and happiness.

"Fuck, I'm in love!" she said loudly after she closed the door behind him.

Two days later, she ran into Bailey at work. "OMG Amelia, I must talk to you. Let's have lunch. Or can I come to your office?" Her desire to meet seemed urgent, so Amelia agreed to welcome her into her office the next day.

The moment she walked in, she started talking, full of energy and excitement. "You know I'm in love with a man who is much older than me. He is smart, and I love his company. But he's also confusing me. You know he works for our company, and I don't know if I should keep seeing him," said Bailey. "He's also terrible with texting. He travels all the time and doesn't reply for days. Then he bombards me with messages. I'm confused. Is this what men do?"

"What does he look like? How old is he?" Amelia asked curiously.

"Why does it matter? I want you to help me! Should I be fucking a man who is twenty-five years older than me and works in the same department?"

"You must decide. It can create problems. When did you see him last?"

"He came to the company networking event two days ago. I was almost gone; it was way past nine o'clock when I saw him arriving with the biggest smile on his face. Oh, he is so charming. Apparently, he had tons of work, but I would imagine he was with another woman—he looked so happy and satisfied. We flirted and got drunk, and he ended up at my house. We tried to have sex, but he was very tired, so we made out. He woke up early and left for the airport. Now he has been texting me all day about whether I'm OK and when he can see me next!"

She kept talking about him, but Amelia didn't hear anything more. Her ears were ringing, and her head was spinning. There were too many signs. But she couldn't believe it. Thinking about her looks, her elegance, her sexuality and brains, and then looking at her colleague, who was cute, but...she was so different from Amelia, and young enough to be his daughter. *No, it can't be him. He is way too sexy and definitely has a higher bar.* What the heck was she thinking? *Stop!* she told herself and smiled, but she was dying to know more about him. Just in case.

"So how long has this been going on?" asked Amelia again.

"About a couple of months. We have been texting and seeing each other every now and then. He always comes to my house. Oh gosh, is he a good lover! But so tall, my Eduard!" Bailey smiled, and Amelia felt a rush of blood all over her body and had to sip some water so as not to pass out.

It's a sad and quite unbelievable story. I felt bad for Amelia, and it took her a while to recover. "But he wasn't her boyfriend," you might say. I know, but when you experience such a deep connection with someone and you're infatuated for months, this shit hurts. And why do many men act this way and not want to commit to monogamy even if they have great sex and a deep connection with someone? What are the reasons why many women struggle to get men to agree to a serious relationship, and for many, it's a seemingly impossible mission? Why do women get attached more quickly than men and want to sleep around less?

There are many answers to this question. Some researchers believe that natural factors such as differences in the brain's structure and activity, hormonal release, and the challenges of reproduction (women's high cost of creating offspring versus men's low cost) contribute to differentiating men's approach from that of women. Others argue that those behaviors are shifting through the influence of culture and upbringing. Even though the trend for women today is to embrace their sexual desires and urges, women must grapple with the natural instinct of wanting to form a bond with a male partner, even if there are no offspring as a result of sexual activity. Or perhaps, women would have to get over the fear and shame that was forced on them for so many years in order to behave more like men in matters of sex. So, is it nature or nurture that influences male and female behaviors around casual sex and hookups?

NEUROBIOLOGY

I always wondered whether the female brain is different from the male brain and if that is why many women can't act the same way men do when it comes to sex. The brain is a mosaic of male and female characteristics. No brain is entirely male or entirely female. The differences in the brain can predict certain behaviors, but the newest research has proven that the brain is no more gendered than the heart or liver or kidney.[31] The biggest physiological difference is

---

[31] Richard J. Haier, Rex E. Jung, Ronald A. Yeo, Kevin Head, and Michael T. Alkire, "The Neuroanatomy of General Intelligence: Sex Matters," *NeuroImage* 25, no. 1 (March 2005): 320–27, https://doi.org/10.1016/j.neuroimage.2004.11.019.

the size: proportional to body size, not influencing how intelligent one is. (In other words, men aren't smarter than women; they reach the same levels of IQ but through a collaboration of different brain parts. Sorry, gentlemen!)

Research about the brain via functional magnetic resonance imaging (fMRI) studies has identified a number of differences in aspects of sexual behavior between men and women. In one experiment,[32] twenty-eight adults, fourteen women and fourteen men, were shown sexy nude pictures of the opposite gender and a picture of a couple having sex. Men showed much greater activity in the amygdala and hypothalamus, even though women reported higher arousal. The amygdala and hypothalamus are parts of the limbic brain, the most primitive part of our brain that mainly controls emotions, survival instincts, and fear. Sex is a survival instinct, as humans are made to procreate. This means men are basically just trying to save humanity by fucking as many women as possible—which is likely why it's easier for men to sleep around and why it takes less for them to get turned on than it does for women.

As Ogas and Gaddam suggest in their book[33] *A Billion Wicked Thoughts*, "Men's greater sex drive may be partially due to the fact that

---

32 Stephan Hamann, Rebecca A Herman, Carla L Nolan, and Kim Wallen, "Men and Women Differ in Amygdala Response to Visual Sexual Stimuli," Nature Neuroscience 7, no. 4 (March 7, 2004): 411–16, https://doi.org/10.1038/nn1208.

33 Ogi Ogas and Sai Gaddam, *A Billion Wicked Thoughts: What the Internet Tells Us About Sexual Relationships* (New York: Plume, 2012).

their sexual motivation pathways have more connections to the sub-cortical reward system than in women." The term *subcortical reward system* describes a group of brain structures that become activated by rewarding or reinforcing stimuli, in this case seeing an attractive woman, naked body parts, legs, breasts, and so on. In short, it means that men are born to objectify women. Staring at women creates a "sex-like" experience, and men's brains will release that feel-good chemical. There is nothing we can do about this, and it explains why men need just a little bit to get turned on and have sex. Once the good feeling is over, they have a tendency to move on to another target.

For women, the sexual motivation pathways are not as close to the reward system. Therefore, we usually don't get turned on by getting another dick pic. (Men, pay attention: unless the woman you're into asks for a dick pic, *do not* send one. I got so many dick pics over the course of my life that at some point I wanted to create a giant collage from the hundreds of dick pics I had collected and invite all the guys who sent them to me for the exhibition debut. There I'd encourage them to find their own penis out of the hundreds.) Women need more context to get aroused. The cliché that men like sexy outfits and lingerie and women like to be wined and dined and have a titillating conversation has been scientifically proven.

EVOLUTION

There are two types of reproductive strategies, the first of which is having tons of kids and not taking care of them at all. This is seen in numerous fish species, some of which have thousands of offspring but don't care for them—they just leave them to live or die on their own. The idea here is that some will manage to survive, and some always do. The other strategy, seen for example in elephants (and other mammals), is to have fewer offspring but to take better care of them.

Now, human men, if left to their own devices, would likely lean more toward the fish strategy. Remember, though, that female reproductive strategies drive the bus, and human females utilize the elephant strategy. Thus, it is the female strategy that moderates male behavior. Now, females need to ensure the survival of their offspring (and that benefits men too), so through the approximately seven million years of bipedal (upright walking) evolution, our species has evolved a number of strategies to help ensure the survival of offspring.

One of those strategies involves strong, emotional, familial bonds. Another strategy we've developed is living in cultural groups. With regard to the first strategy, familial bonds, humans are a species with a polygynous evolutionary history. "Poly" means many, and "gyny" means women. The higher reproductive potential and low cost of reproduction for male humans make men more sexually eager than female humans, whose reproductive potential is limited and comes at a greater energetic cost. It takes much more energy to gestate a baby, and then nurse it and keep it alive after it is born, than it does to engage in one sexual act. Therefore, females are naturally more choosy concerning mates and mating. And that's why the females evolved to form strong, emotional, familial bonds with the males and also with female relatives, who could help them raise the offspring at least to approximately four years of age, when the child becomes physically and mentally able to assist in his or her own survival. In other words, he/she can understand and obey if Mom says, "go hide" or "run." Having the help of a group invested in the child's survival is why most evolutionary scientists believe polygynous groups—that is, groups composed of one male or just a few males, and several more females—became a successful female reproductive strategy.

The theory is that early human ancestors likely formed groups of a few males and several females. The males would protect the group from danger as well as help care for the offspring, and of course, mate with the females. The females would form bonds with (typically) related females who would assist the males in protecting the group as necessary and care for the offspring.

This has several beneficial effects. Having several females helping you raise your offspring allows you to recover from the birth process and be ready to have more babies more rapidly than if you didn't have help. It is also evolutionarily advantageous for females to care for the offspring of related females. If you're an aunt, it is to your genetic advantage—your "fitness"—to care for your nieces and nephews. They carry some of your genes—remember, "the fittest" is defined by how many genes you leave on the planet. Therefore, related females benefit from helping their relatives' offspring survive, and those aunts who care for their nieces and nephews get valuable experience in raising offspring by doing so. When it comes time to have their own children, they are better prepared to be good mothers.

Males also benefit from this strategy, given that they can produce more of their own offspring, and those offspring are more likely to survive. Therefore, biological anthropologists and other evolutionary scientists agree that rearing our children as a team—"it takes a village" —gave us an edge for survival. But living in a group setting, as our species does, requires establishing a set of rules. For our species, that meant the evolution of culture, which, as we'll discuss below, has a significant effect on behavior.

Fast-forward a few million years to between 5,000 and 7,000 years ago. Now, we have fully modern humans having large-brained infants and living in complex hierarchical cultural groups. In this environment, it became more advantageous to form monogamous bonds, as this allowed for the formation of stronger alliances between various groups and families. In that context, women benefit from a monogamous union, given that all of the man's resources are focused on her and her offspring; she doesn't have to share his resources with other women and their children.

The man also benefits, because he can be more certain that any children born of that union are his. It is far easier to control access (of other males) to one female than it is to several females. He is, therefore, more motivated to care for the offspring, something that also benefits his partner. Considering this fact, it makes sense that after a sexual experience, even if a woman isn't pregnant and awaiting her offspring, she's hardwired to need the man to stick around for her survival. This explains our biological attachment and cravings for the male after a casual hookup.

In fact, female biology is geared toward keeping the man around. Evolutionary scientists believe that this may be the reason behind the switch to the menstrual cycle rather than the estrous cycle that most other mammalian animals have. With the menstrual cycle, there's no visible indicator that a female is receptive to mating. In other words, the man has no visible way of knowing when a woman is most likely to become pregnant. This is in contrast to the estrous cycle, where the female genitalia swell and become red, something the male can see (and smell) as an indicator that the female is sexually receptive and ovulating. The estrous cycle is seen in horses, sheep, goats, deer, cats, dogs, and others. Human females have no such signal, and therefore, a man has to woo a woman, and he usually has to mate with her several times to produce offspring—yes, it can happen after only one time, but usually it takes more.

In fact, it takes, on average, one hundred times before pregnancy results. That's due in part to the fact that there is, relatively speaking, a wide timeframe in which the woman may be ovulating, as opposed to the estrous cycle where the female is ovulating only during the short time when she's bleeding. A human woman is ovulating at some point in the approximately twenty-one days when she is not bleeding. Therefore, the "fittest" men stick around long enough to produce offspring, by which time they've likely formed an emotional bond with the female. That causes them to also want to contribute to ensuring the survival of those offspring, and that ultimately makes them more "fit."

Given the realities of human biology, honed through millions of years of evolution and tempered by human culture, it's not surprising that women respond with anxiety when they mate with a man and he then disappears. A rational mind doesn't help much when pitted against survival instincts that are controlled through our limbic brain. Moreover, like human biology, human culture has evolved to manipulate sexual behaviors so as to encourage monogamous unions, particularly where female sexuality is concerned. In fact, as monogamous unions became the norm, it became critical to control female sexual behavior. If you're a king who wants to form an alliance with another country, you might do so by having your daughter marry that king's son. But, if your daughter is "tainted" because she is not a virgin, it will be more difficult to make that deal. Your daughter's virginity is vital to your own power.

It was within the context of controlling female sexuality for these kinds of purposes that women came to be viewed as the property of men, either their father's or their husband's. And, as their property, women were forced to be what the mainstream culture identified as virtuous. This forced women to act in ways contrary to their own biology, their own natural desires, and their own instincts.

CULTURE AND UPBRINGING

Nature versus nurture is an age-old question. When it comes to sex, researchers have done some interesting studies to find out how much of our sexual behavior is due to our genes and how much is because of the way we are nurtured. To find out more, they used identical twins for their experiments. The results were quite interesting. Thirty-four percent of us inherited the age of our first intercourse and 46 percent of other sexual behaviors.[34] You might wonder how on earth you could inherit the age of your first intercourse, right? Well, the participants reported the same age of first intercourse as their parents did. When it comes to other sexual behaviors, it means that the parents reported a non-monogamous lifestyle. This might mean that if our parents have a monogamous sex life, there's almost a half chance that we will have the same life.

But what if we see other behaviors in our peers and friends? This study shows that the rest of our sexual behaviors are controlled by

---

[34] K. Paige Harden, "Genetic Influences on Adolescent Sexual Behavior: Why Genes Matter for Environmentally Oriented Researchers," *Psychological Bulletin* 140, no. 2 (2014): 434–65, https://doi.org/10.1037/a0033564.

non-genetic factors such as individual psychological makeup, childhood experiences, and culture. Culture is all human-cultivated behavior. That refers to the entirety of a person's learned, accumulated experiences, which are socially transmitted. It is not biological. As you grow up, you're taught a value system supported and encouraged by the culture in which you live. Only very rarely, relatively speaking, will you question that value system. Most people simply accept it and live their lives in accordance with those values.

There are also rebels out there who will question what is right and what is wrong. They'll ask why things are a certain way, and they won't accept the given norm. Already, as little babies, we are subconsciously listening to our parents, grandparents, and other family members saying and showing what is right and wrong. Admonishments like "boys don't cry" and "girls must be cute and quiet" will stick with you forever.

When it comes to sex, there have been a number of studies that have documented cultural double standards regarding sexual behavior in men and women. Whereas men, particularly young men, are encouraged to desire and pursue sexual relations regardless of emotional or relational context, women are permitted to engage in sexual relations only in the context of true love and a committed relationship.[35] This has a long and complicated history and, as discussed, has been

---

[35] Mary Crawford and Danielle Popp, "Sexual Double Standards: A Review and Methodological Critique of Two Decades of Research," *Journal of Sex Research* 40, no. 1 (February 2003): 13–26, https://doi.org/10.1080/00224490309552163.

perpetuated by every major religion. Even Confucianism viewed female chastity as a virtue, and while male chastity was seen as a high goal, it was also seen as mainly unattainable. Thus, sons are encouraged to sow their wild oats, while a daughter is expected to be a virgin when she reaches the altar.

Those who espouse these views don't seem bothered by the internal inconsistencies. With whom are the boys supposed to "be boys," if the girls are to remain chaste? In the past, when women violated their chastity, they were subjected to status loss and discrimination. In my case, in mid-1990s post-communistic Slovakia, I paid for my early exploration by being shamed and bullied. After doing all this research, I confirmed what I already knew: that men are not the only ones who use "slut-shaming" to enforce perceived cultural norms and exert dominance.

In marriage, the same rules apply in terms of the monogamy that is considered a norm in our culture, and everything besides that is considered dirty or unacceptable. This is because non-monogamy is foreign to many people in our culture. Usually, we don't understand things that are foreign to us. Not only that, but what we don't understand, we are scared and judgmental of. It's a natural reaction that I have observed in so many people. Sadly, the idea of accepting whatever has been thought of as normal and judging anything that's new to us without exploring and doing our own research, leads to prejudice and hatred.

CONTEMPORARY FACTORS

B esides nature and nurture, there are other factors that make people behave non-monogamously around sex and leave most men unwilling to commit. Some are technological. Others are because of the fear of missing out (FOMO), which is so prevalent in younger generations and related to social media. Lastly, others are due to the financial challenges of the millennial generation.

Swipe right, swipe left

Apps such as Tinder or Fling make it easy to swipe and have a one-night stand, so why would any man bother to invest quality time in one particular match? Through the false perception of unlimited choices and abundance, a man can come to believe there is a line of women waiting for him. He might think, "Why would I settle for Jane when I'm also chatting with Jessica and Susan, and they're both available tomorrow?"

Men as well as women in the millennial generation are overwhelmed with choices, and not just when it comes to dating and choosing the right partner. Traveling has become more accessible due to travel apps that search for the cheapest flights and hotels. We also have endless overpriced educational possibilities online. We can get any credit card we want with a credit limit much higher than what we can actually afford. We can rent clothing, jewelry, electronics, and apartments and swap them at any time. The days when people would purchase a home and live there for decades are over. Most millennials don't even own their homes, and if they do, they often share them; the same is true of their cars. Why would we buy something for a longer term when we can literally create a new home and a new experience every year, exchange our wardrobe on a monthly basis, and travel to a new destination every other weekend?

The number of choices we have is making us not want to commit. Committing to one partner (or car, or apartment, or wardrobe) seems too scary. Not only that, but why would we when there are so many great things out there waiting for us?

But are so many choices actually good for our happiness and satisfaction?

One study[36] shows that this plethora of choices can lead to a "choice overload" phenomenon. This study examined the satisfaction of people who had limited choices—in this case, six—as opposed to those who had a greater number of options (between twenty-four and thirty). It found that those who had more options were actually more dissatisfied with their choice as well as being more confused in their decision-making process than those whose options were limited. And exactly the same thing happens in the realm of dating and hookups. We can meet so many potential partners that before

---

[36] Sheena S. Iyengar and Mark R. Lepper, "When Choice Is Demotivating: Can One Desire Too Much of a Good Thing?" *Journal of Personality and Social Psychology* 79, no. 6 (December 2000): 995–1006, https://doi.org/10.1037/0022-3514.79.6.995.

we can truly enjoy one, pay attention to the moment, and try to get to know them, we're already thinking about whom we will reach out to next. After ten dates where we still don't find the right one and connect on a deeper level, we begin feeling empty and dissatisfied, thinking something is wrong with us!

In my early thirties, when I was single and living in Manhattan, I dated Nicholas. We met through friends and liked each other immediately. At first sight, he was a perfect catch. I could check all the basic boxes: young, successful, good-looking, fairly affluent, with a promising career and an excellent education. He sounds like a dream, doesn't he? We moved into intense dating very quickly, since he was looking for a girlfriend as well—at least that's what I heard from his best friend, who was dating my roommate back then. Shortly after our first date, I spent the weekend at his place, and then he spent the weekend at my place. We spoke on the phone twice a week, and he replied to my messages in a timely fashion. "What a great guy he is, and so sexy!" I thought. I smiled every evening while reading his messages.

We kept up this pace for about two months and then decided to go on our first vacation to the Caribbean. It was the middle of January, and we both needed some sun. The very first day, when we were lying on the beach, I realized how much time he spent on his phone. I thought he must be dealing with some work, so I let him be. It wasn't minutes —it was hours. I got no attention or conversation that entire day. And to make things worse, he did the same thing in restaurants, bars, and for the next two days on the beach. I was getting very impatient, as

I had many friends vacationing at the same location and wanted to see them. I felt that I was wasting my time with this man, since all of his attention was given to his cell phone. I got nothing!

On the third day, as we sat at the dinner table, my patience ran out. We ordered some food and drinks, and once again, he started looking at his phone under the table rather than carrying on any sort of conversation with me. I felt so awkward and angry at that point that I quickly stood up, walked around the table, and grabbed his phone out of his hand. "What the fuck are you looking at all the time? This is so disrespectful!" I yelled at him and looked at the phone.

I know that he probably thought I was crazy and that he would never see me again after this trip, but I didn't care because I felt the same way. I just wanted to know what the heck was so important that he had to spend hours doing it under the table and on the beach and in our bed while we were on vacation. I basically needed that "he's an asshole" confirmation so I could move on without any regrets. And I got it.

Quite frankly, I thought he was texting with another woman. But no! He was on Tinder, swiping right and left, looking at what he could find out there in the wild. He was, in fact, texting with many women, trying to convince them to come and surprise us in the hotel for a threesome. Holy moly! This was a real shock for me. And I thought I'd seen it all! When I asked him what the hell made him think that would be a good idea, he said that he thought he couldn't satisfy me enough, and since he also knew about my bisexual tendencies, he wanted to surprise me! Whatever. As you can imagine, our relationship was over.

This is exactly what I'm talking about when it comes to all the dating apps and social media. We don't live in the moment, get to know each other better, pay attention to who the other person really is, listen and learn about each other; instead, we are focusing on what's next. And social media only makes it worse.

Empirical research[37] has actually shown that a significant number of people using mobile dating apps are already in a committed relationship. The reasons why they're looking to be unfaithful to their partner are varied, but the point is that hooking up with them isn't likely to lead to a committed relationship. Thus, it appears that while singles using dating apps may well be hoping to eventually find a committed relationship, as many as 40 percent of US users of dating apps are simply looking to have an affair. That suggests they have a lower level of commitment to their steady relationship and would presumably be less likely to remain committed in a new relationship as well. Researchers have also found that willingness to commit to a longer-term relationship among mobile dating app users was dependent on the number of dating options available to the user. The more options they had, the less likely they were to commit.

---

[37] Cassandra Alexopoulos, Elisabeth Timmermans, and Jenna McNallie, "Swiping More, Committing Less: Unraveling the Links among Dating App Use, Dating App Success, and Intention to Commit Infidelity," *Computers in Human Behavior* 102 (January 2020): 172–80, https://doi.org/10.1016/j.chb.2019.08.009.

Likewise, researchers found that the use of mobile dating apps provided individuals in a committed relationship with a spontaneous and frequent source of temptation for hooking up. That made it more difficult for them to maintain their relationship given that they were constantly reminded of the amount and quality of any other users that were within their proximity. The same study also found that the number of available partners and self-perceived desirability of mobile dating app users was positively correlated with an intention to commit infidelity. Essentially, if you perceive yourself as desirable and you have a higher number of potential hookups in your area, you're more likely to go for it! That may be good for you, but it's not great for your committed relationship.

What does this mean for you? If you're in a committed relationship and don't want to screw things up, do not install a dating app. Not only is it inappropriate, but it can create irresistible desire.

FOMO:
The Fear of Missing Out

A while ago, I was interviewed about the influence of social media on romantic relationships. As you might assume, and perhaps know for yourself, through the impact of social media, you may suffer from a serious case of FOMO. You want to experience more partners, more travel, and more fun, and this will also keep you from feeling satisfied with one partner in the long run. There are so many pretty faces and half-naked bodies online that often men would rather spend their time clicking "like" on Instagram or Twitter than sending a polite text to the hookup partner they had last night. FOMO makes people constantly look for the bigger and better thing rather than appreciating what they already have.

Social media also creates a false sense of reality about female faces and bodies that are mostly retouched and adjusted with beauty apps, which might set a high bar for the physical beauty of the women that men would like to date. These "avatar"-looking pictures of half-naked ladies on Instagram create the fantasy that many men then try to fulfill on Tinder and other dating apps. But women like that do not exist. Even the prettiest women I know look different in real life than on their Instagram posts. Women, after a whole night of sex, do not look like avatars!

Social media also contributes to the feeling that we can never meet the perfect partner with whom we can have a magical connection. The romance seen on TV screens and under hashtags like #relationshipgoals or #couplesgoals is not easily achieved. These posts portray amazing relationships, ultimate connections, and eternal happiness, something so unachievable for us humans that we would rather give up if things aren't perfect than put any sort of effort and dedication into building a solid relationship.

But, besides the simplicity of hooking up these days through technology and social media, it is the phenomena of too many choices and FOMO that are keeping many of us from building long-term bonds. And there's one other important factor in why people are scared of commitments: financial concerns.

No Money, No Honey
(Or, Why Millennials are Basically Fucked)

Many millennials choose not to marry and have children because of existential difficulties. Get ready for some hardcore statistics, which I'm about to share. (And get a tissue because what I've learned is truly sad.)

One in five millennials lives in poverty[38]—that's 20 percent. Millennials are about half as likely to own a home as young adults were in 1975; they have taken on 300 percent more student debt than their parents did, and most millennials simply won't be able to retire until they are over seventy-five years old. While many members of older generations tend to think that millennials are a bunch of entitled babies, the truth is that the world is a much different place for them than it was for earlier generations.[39] While wages have stagnated, entire sectors of the economy have cratered, and the 2008 recession hit millennials harder than any other age group. Moreover, the cost of

---

[38] "The Millennial Generation Research Review," *U.S. Chamber of Commerce Foundation*, last modified November 12, 2012, https://www.uschamberfoundation.org/reports/millennial-generation-research-review.

[39] Kristen Bialik and Richard Fry, "Millennial Life: How Young Adulthood Today Compares with Prior Generations," *Pew Research Center*, last modified January 30, 2019, https://www.pewsocial trends.org/essay/millennial-life-how-young-adulthood-today-compares-with-prior-generations/.

pretty much everything that helps create a secure existence—things like education, homeownership, and healthcare—has soared. This is occurring at the same time that social safety nets are eroding. Basically, a perfect storm designed to fuck millennials has been forming for years, and it is only now making landfall.

The situation has created the one thing that truly defines the millennial generation: uncertainty. Consider the fact that in 2007, more than 50 percent of seniors graduating from college already had a job offer lined up. By 2009, less than 20 percent did. Also, a soaring unemployment rate equates with significant drops in starting salaries. In fact, just a 1 percent rise in the unemployment rate corresponds to a 6 to 8 percent drop in starting salaries.

Now, consider that millennials suffered one blow in 2008 and have been hit with another with the COVID-19 recession. Talk about piling on! That's two disadvantages that will have lasting effects that can linger in an individual's life for decades to come. Added to these problems is the fact that millennials are unable to participate in parts of the economy, like homeownership, that offer them the opportunity to build generational wealth.[40] Homeownership by people between the ages of twenty-five and thirty-four peaked at 47 percent in 2005. The housing market crisis that followed in 2007 resulted in a decrease

---

[40] Jung Choi, "Homeownership and Living Arrangements Among Millennials: New Sources of Wealth Inequality and What to Do about It," *New America*. accessed November 14, 2020, https://www.newamerica.org/millennials/reports/emerging-millennial-wealth-gap/homeownership-and-living-arrangements-among-millennials-new-sources-of-wealth-inequality-and-what-to-do-about-it/.

to 37 percent in 2015. If the millennials in this age group had the same rate of homeownership as their 2000- era cohorts, the result would be 1.3 million more young homeowners in the United States.

When you consider the benefits of homeownership in generating sustainable wealth, this is a significant problem for millennials. But why aren't millennials buying houses? The answer is simple: real estate is ridiculously expensive. Many millennials have to live in downtown areas due to work opportunities, and housing there is far from affordable. Access to credit has tightened since the 2008 recession, and of course, millennials also have lower incomes and higher student debt.[41]

Knowing all of this, how could one feel safe and confident enough to date seriously? Love and long-term relationships usually lead to marriage, with the potential of having a family. A family needs a decent home. So why are millennials postponing marriage and having a family? Because they simply can't afford it![42]

I hope I didn't ruin all your dreams about good relationships. They definitely exist. I shared this with you simply to explain where a male's head often is when he is difficult and doesn't want to commit. You might catch yourself having this problem, too. Some suggestions on

---

[41] Megan Leonhardt, "Millennials Earn 20% Less Than Baby Boomers Did—Despite Being Better Educated," *CNBC*, last modified November 5, 2019, https://www.cnbc.com/2019/11/05/millennials-earn-20-percent-less-than-boomersdespite-being-better-educated.html.

[42] Michael Hobbes, "FML: Why Millennials are Facing the Scariest Financial Future of Any Generation Since the Great Depression," *The Huffington Post*, accessed May 12, 2021,. https://highline.huffingtonpost.com/articles/en/poor-millennials/.

how to fight FOMO are to stop swiping through online dating apps, live more in the present moment, and enjoy your surroundings and the people you know instead of seeking new ones. If you meet a beau you like, give him a chance and get to know him better. Maybe you'll find some good qualities and then will want to spend more time with him than with your fantasy men.

What about when it comes to the men you're dating? I hate to tell you this, but when a man isn't ready to commit to you after you've been seeing him for some time and have been honest about your feelings, there are only two solutions to this problem. One is that you can try all possible seduction techniques to get him to fall in love with you and commit to you. This route can cost you a lot of energy and time, and you might or might not be successful. Before you start, please make sure he is worth it: learn as much as you can about him, his family, work, and habits, so you're aware of what you are actually investing your time and effort into. On how to seduce him and make him fall in love with you, I have no easy answer. Techniques change from man to man. I'd probably need another book on this topic, but one of the best books I've read about seduction and how to make men fall in love with you is *The Art of Seduction* by Robert Greene. Check it out and learn from there.

My second piece of advice is to realize that after a while, if he isn't into more than just occasional sex, you might just call it a day and find someone else. If a man isn't able to deal with FOMO, he might not be grown-up enough to even have a serious relationship. If he's still using dating apps after he has met you, he isn't that impressed with you, and you should move on unless you're OK with being his sex object and having him as yours.

I truly believe in love magic, and once you meet the one, you both will feel it and forget all the other ones out there. He will stop looking at the apps and social media and enjoy you for you. I believe things that unfold organically are the best and longest lasting. I know some women who spent a ton of time fighting for men they were in love with. They spent years seducing these men and trying to get them to marry. Some of them succeeded, but many did only for the short term. Even when they married and had babies, these men were internally dissatisfied and felt trapped or pushed into the marriage. Men love to hunt, and if they can't chase the woman and try to "get" her, she might feel too easy to get for them. Men tend to not value something they get too easily. Many of these unhappy men, with their FOMO and non-monogamous tendencies, ended up cheating anyway. So make sure that doesn't happen to you, and don't chase him too hard. Even if you do, it must look like it's coming from him. He must be the one chasing you and getting you to marry him. You must be his victory.

What about the solution to the financial issues? As I said, do your research. Find out about his job and background. I'm not suggesting you have to only date a man who has money, but he should at least have a job and not be sinking in debt. Debt stress doesn't help the relationship, and you don't want to be solving his financial issues. If he, as they say, has his shit together, go for it. Because when you love each other, you'll be able to collectively create a better lifestyle.

PLAYERS AND THEIR COACHES

We've all encountered a player or ten in our lives, right? They are fun, but they can make your life hell if you fall in love with them. That's why I put together a list of characteristics to help you recognize them so you can avoid them—or only use them for your pleasure, if you're a "coach."

How to recognize a player

Who's a player? This term is mostly used for a man who is faking his serious interest in a relationship and romance. Oftentimes, a player, with his lies and pretense, can trick you into thinking that he's looking for commitment. But he can't pretend for too long, and soon you'll see his real face.

Why do players try to deceive us? Why can't they be honest and say they just want to play around? Because telling the truth would decrease their chances for hookups. Most women don't like the idea of being just a casual fling, and they hope for a romance and more commitment. It's much easier for a player to deceive a woman in order to get laid. Some players need constant masturbation of their egos. They're proud of their "skills" with women, the knowledge they have about women and, crudely, about their partner count. There are also a small number of players who want to hurt and punish women because of their past traumas with exes, mothers, or sisters. Beware of them!

How can you identify these men? And if you do catch one, what should you do with him? The second question is easy, in my mind: if you have a casual-sex mindset and he's good-looking and flirtatious, have sex and never call him again. When he's the player, you'll be the coach! The first question is a little more complicated, so let me share a game plan with you. Look out for the following characteristics and you'll be able to identify a player in a second:

1. A player will not remember the details of your conversation. Most of them are egocentric and narcissistic, and all they care about is their own pleasure. Although he'll pretend that he's listening, nodding and looking into your eyes, he won't remember the exact details you shared with him. Information about your work, your siblings, and how your boss is a stressful cunt will not remain in his brain. But he'll remember your perky hips and the skirt you wore last time for sure.

2. When talking to a player, you won't be able to have a meaningful and deep conversation. It's just not his style, and in his mind, those are reserved for close friends or committed partners. He will not ask about your family, your work, or anything that could slightly make you feel closer to him or require him to look like he'd care. He

will keep talking about unimportant things, leading you in small talk, talking about travels and fancy things, and mix it with an endless number of compliments about your looks and clothing. Many players have low self-esteem and will talk a lot. Even if he asks you a question, he will interrupt you quickly before you can fully answer and will begin to talk about himself again.

3. A player will try to impress you with superficial and obvious things, such as money, business success, or people he knows—pretty much anything material, because players do not have many other values and disregard the importance of kindness, honesty, and support. I'm not saying all players are terrible people, but they're definitely dishonest and superficial.

4. A player will pressure you heavily to come to his house or let him come to yours. He will be upset if you won't sleep with him or if you refuse his invitation, because that's a terrible defeat for his ego. A player doesn't have the patience to try to persuade you for too long and wants quick gratification.

5. A player will not plan ahead. He'll call you at the last minute or at awkward times, and especially on days when most of us make plans in advance (e.g., late evenings, Sunday afternoons, etc.). This shows you that his first or

second date probably fell through and he's bored, going through a list of potential booty calls to see who is available. Most likely he sent out this message to five of you. If you reply and he doesn't get back to you, you can be sure that his rule is first come, first served.

6. A player won't hold your hand in public or show any sort of intimacy. He avoids public displays of affection (PDA) whenever possible. Don't confuse PDA with a long, juicy French kiss on the way to his house or some touching and grabbing after a couple of glasses of wine. Consider this your foreplay. The moment you get to his house, he will want quick action, and your orgasm won't be his priority.

7. A player won't listen to your sorrow, pain, or anything negative. When you start talking about something personal, he'll quickly derail the conversation and change the topic to food, weather, and sex. A player isn't interested in your private life. The communication he provides will be full of compliments, flirting, and easy topics, with a focus on hooking up, as that's all he's interested in.

8. A player will do anything to flatter you. He will be sweet and give you many superficial compliments that center on your looks, clothing, and body parts. "You have long legs, I'm sure they go to heaven." Sometimes they will overdo it with compliments and will be overly sweet and attentive

without even knowing you. I have learned that when things are too good to be true, they usually are.

9. A player will call you "babe," "hon," "sugar," "sexy," etc. Anything but your name. It's safer to call all women by one name, as there's less chance to confuse them and make a mistake.

10. A player will try to avoid conversations about love, romance, and relationships. There are men and women who aren't ready for a committed relationship, but when they're honest with you, you have a choice of whether to stick around or go. Since the sole purpose of a player is to have sex and leave, or lie to obtain more possible sexual interactions, he will omit his real goals, deceive you, and derail this conversation at all costs.

11. When a player is fishing, he usually hangs out alone or goes out with one or, maximum, two guy friends in order to keep his "real" life a secret. He won't introduce you to his friends, even if you spend more time with him. He doesn't want you to invade his private circle and perhaps find out things about him. When you pay close attention, you might see him showing pictures of the women he slept with in recent days or weeks to his friends while you're close by, much like my short-term friend in Miami with his creepy gallery of Polaroids.

12. A player will most likely ask you to send him a nude picture for his collection. Once you send it, he'll ask for a more provocative one, or even a video of you masturbating! Don't do that! Your picture will circle around.

13. A player will most likely send you a dick pic. He thinks his cock is unique and impeccable, and he'll want to share his treasure with you before you hook up. He could potentially send you some pictures of him in a nice car, on a jet (it's rarely his), or from first class on an airplane. You could also receive pictures of him having drinks in a fancy bar, making sure you see the bottle of Dom Perignon in the background.

14. A player won't spend time on foreplay or care about your pleasure. Forget about massage or oral sex. He wants to go straight to sex. And if you ask him to do these things with you, he will do them for approximately two minutes before he'll get annoyed and enter your vagina. Maybe a good trick to make him work and get rid of him is to tell him to massage you and lick you until orgasm before he can play. My hunch is that he won't be able to do it, as he doesn't have the patience and skills to make you come. If he does, you can choose to get tired and leave or reward him with your vagina. Up to you!

Part 4

. . . .

FOR MEN

Either you made it this far in my book, or perhaps you chose to read only this chapter. In any case, I'm glad you're here. Here, I'll give you some tips on how to help women deal with the post-hookup madness that is caused by biology and culture. It's quite fascinating to know about how we got from having orgies, living in the trees, and following a rule that "sharing is caring" to a lifestyle characterized by monogamy, jealousy, and greed. (You can find all the info on those things in Part 3 of this book.) But since you're here, I assume that you care about female happiness and want to have a smooth ending to your casual endeavors. Sure, you can choose not to reply, to ghost, or to lie —but that won't make women feel any better. Plus, negative energy will be sent your way. Don't forget, what goes around comes around.

To lay everything out on the table, there's not a lot of research into the topic of how to treat a woman post-hookup. As I'm sure you know, though, there are plenty of anecdotal and common-sense suggestions for how to handle the situation. First, if you do want to see her again but you are really busy, don't text her about it. That will probably give her the wrong idea. Instead, call her and tell her that you are interested in getting to know her better, but you are truly super busy. Let her know that you would like to find time for a date in the near future, but you'll have to check your schedule and send her a few possibilities. Then, do what you said you would do!

The trickier situation, however, is if you've hooked up with her and you really don't want to see her again. What do you do then, particularly if she's contacting you? How do you let her down with class? Informal surveys of men and women have resulted in a few good suggestions and some great insight. First, all women hate ghosting …you know, when you just ignore her? Remember, this is a person, and you might have had some great sex together. Show her a little respect. Aside from not ghosting her, here are a few other tips to let her down easy:

1. If you've seen each other a couple of times, it's always nice to reach out, even if just for talking or tea. That way you can tell her to her face that you don't feel a romantic connection with her. This will make her feel appreciated even though you're saying you don't want to see her romantically anymore. If you've only hooked up once,

it might not be necessary to get together in person. Again, though, even if you decide to text her, be respectful.

2. Don't convince yourself that she can't handle it. Women are much stronger than men might think. We are capable of handling some very difficult challenges in life, so be ready to simply state how you feel. She can take it.

3. Sandwich your rejection with compliments. There must be some qualities you liked about her, and letting her know those will help to soften the bad news. It's also helpful if you can break the tension with specific, humorous moments from your hookup. That lets her know that you were in the moment while you were with her. It also helps smooth over telling her that you're just not that into her. For example, maybe she talked too much about herself and didn't seem interested in learning about you. You might say something like, "I'm so impressed by all you've accomplished in your life, and anyone would be lucky to spend more time with you. For me, though, I just didn't feel the kind of connection I'm looking for in a long-term relationship."

4. Be upfront about your feelings. Most women are accustomed to almost constantly analyzing and dissecting men's behavior. It's an exhausting and often tormenting process, and it would be a lot easier if you would just be

upfront about your feelings. If you're not interested, just say so. That will let her move on and stop torturing herself with the "what ifs." One woman, when asked about her experiences, noted that she was thankful when a man she had two dates with told her he simply wasn't "feeling" her after the second date. She thanked him and went on with her life. She recalls the experience as the best way to get the news.

5. Don't bother with fake lines, such as that you just want to be friends. Most women prefer clarity and closure. If your hookup partner has questions about why you don't want to see her again, tell her! It's not mean to be upfront about your reasons for not wanting to see her again, but it *is* mean to leave her guessing about what she did wrong. Be kind, be honest, and please keep in mind to tell her the reasons when it comes to differences in personalities and goals or interests. That said, DO NOT criticize her appearance. It can leave a deep scar on someone's ego.

6. Be broad in your reasoning. If she asks why you don't want a second hookup, tell her kindly. You might say something like, "I just feel we have two different approaches to life, and I don't think they're compatible," or "I'm not looking for the same level of commitment as you are." You don't have to put her down, but you need to tell her the truth in as gentle a manner as possible. While

you want to be honest, you don't have to be insulting. Maybe you didn't like the way she was unkind to the waiter or the fact that she seemed too clingy. Instead of hurting her with an insult, you might just say something like "I feel like we have different values" or "I'm someone who needs a lot of space, and I'm not ready to give that up."

7. Don't waste her time. When you lead her on with promises to get together soon, or tell her you'll call her later, you're just keeping her on a string and wasting her time. By clearly telling her you're not interested, you give her the freedom to go look for someone who is. You should never assume she'll get the hint because you're ignoring her. Women have an incredible ability to rationalize your ghosting, so just tell her the truth so she can have closure and move on. It's fine to simply say, "It was nice meeting you, but I just didn't feel a lasting connection. We had some fun, but I don't think it has the potential to develop into anything more serious."

8. Let her know as soon as you can if she's reaching out to you and you know you're not interested. It's best if you can identify what you're feeling. You can say something like, "Hey, this was fun, but I'm not into the second date." Be firm and clear with your intentions. Don't muddy the waters with suggestions that you might do things together

as friends. Just let her know you're moving on and she should too. That's much kinder than giving her any sort of false hope.

9. Take the hints you get from her. Maybe you're into her, but she's just not that into you! A lot of what I'm saying about women is also true for men. If she seems to always be busy or doesn't get back to you, take the hint that maybe she's not interested in a second hookup. If that's the case, move on with your life and let her get on with hers.

10. Keep it respectful, no matter how you choose to let her know. It's best to be honest even though you know it will hurt her feelings. Remember that she is a person with feelings, needs, and dreams, just like you. There's no reason to be cruel or disrespectful. Letting her down in a kind manner will help both of you grow. After all, kindness doesn't cost you a thing.

CONCLUSION

. . . .

Female sexuality is a rich and complex topic. On one hand, we would like to have more fun, hook up easily, and enjoy our sex lives. On the other hand, we're still worried and ashamed to do so. When we finally allow ourselves to have fun, we can fall in love and often end up dealing with discomfort and pain down to our souls. Although we are hardwired for certain behaviors around sex, we *can* change our thinking and start enjoying sex for what it really is—fun and pleasurable. The best part is that we can get rid of all the negative emotions surrounding our sexuality that are so deeply rooted, mainly through culture.

How can we achieve this? First, we must change our way of thinking in order to change our culture. Culture is something that we create on a daily basis. That means we can change it on a daily basis too. The best way is to support cultural elements that are important for healthy sexual expression—for example, providing access to sex education for youth, allowing men and women to express their sexual thoughts and desires freely in a judgment-free environment, and pointing out and discussing the existence of double standards.

As we navigate recent cultural changes regarding sexual behaviors, such as the #MeToo movement, it is clear that women are striving to take control of their own sexual agency. There's real progress in making significant and lasting changes, but lasting change requires the support of women themselves. We have to stop "eating our own." When women unite behind their right to express their sexual desires without attaching stigmas to one another, then men will come around.

Ladies, support each other and wish yourselves as much pleasure as possible. We have a lot to catch up on after all these years! And when you start hooking up, always remember this guide and protect your heart.

Good luck and have fun, no matter what direction you choose.

With love,

Lia

ABOUT THE AUTHOR

Lia Holmgren has been an intimacy and relationship coach for more than a decade, guiding her clients through modern challenges and exploring the many roles of power and fantasy. Known for her empathetic nature and direct style, Lia empowers her clients to feel safe in celebrating their authentic sexuality.

Lia holds an MS in negotiation and conflict resolution from Columbia University and a BS in biopsychology from Touro University. She is a certified wellness coach and life coach as well as a certified hypnotist. Lia has been featured by numerous media outlets, including NBC Universal, *New York Post*, *Huffington Post*, *Men's Health*, *Curtis and Cosy Show*, and more.

liaholmgren.com

CPSIA information can be obtained
at www.ICGtesting.com
Printed in the USA
LVHW010551011021
699182LV00005B/15